# PRIMELIFE PREGNANCY

Also by the author

YOUR PREGNANCY MONTH BY MONTH

# · PRIMELIFE ·
# PREGNANCY

## all you need to know
## about pregnancy after 35

# CLARK GILLESPIE, M.D.

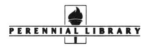

PERENNIAL LIBRARY

HARPER & ROW, PUBLISHERS ○ New York

Cambridge, Philadelphia, San Francisco, Washington
London, Mexico City, São Paulo, Singapore, Sydney

Grateful acknowledgment is made for permission to reprint:

Table on page 20 and chart on page 22 from *Contemporary Ob/Gyn,* April 1984, and statistics on page 107 from *Contemporary Ob/Gyn* 25:117, April 1985.

List on page 19 from American College of Obstetricians and Gynecologists, *Guidelines on Pregnancy and Work* (Washington, D.C.: ACOG, 1977), page 16. Reprinted by permission of the American College of Obstetricians and Gynecologists.

List on page 36 from American College of Obstetricians and Gynecologists, *Exercise During Pregnancy and the Postnatal Period* (ACOG Home Exercise Programs; Washington, D.C.: ACOG, 1985). Reprinted by permission of the American College of Obstetricians and Gynecologists.

Table on page 46 from January–June 1983 *Statistical Bulletin.* Courtesy of Metropolitan Life Insurance Company.

List on pages 70–71 from *Nutrition Action Healthletter.* Reprinted by permission of the Center for Science in the Public Interest.

Table on pages 74–79 from American College of Obstetricians and Gynecologists, *Immunization During Pregnancy,* ACOG Technical Bulletin 64 (Washington, D.C.: ACOG, May 1982). Reprinted by permission of the American College of Obstetricians and Gynecologists.

List on pages 129–30 from American College of Obstetricians and Gynecologists, "IOM Publishes Conclusions on Low Birth Weight," *ACOG Newsletter* 29 (4):5, 1985. Reprinted by permission of the American College of Obstetricians and Gynecologists.

List on page 188 from American College of Obstetricians and Gynecologists, "California Hospital Leads in Number of Births, Averages Nearly 50 a Day," *ACOG Newsletter* 31 (2):11, 1987. Reprinted by permission of the American College of Obstetricians and Gynecologists.

Statistics on pages 274–75 from *The Journal of American Medical Association* 225 (1):76, January 3, 1986. Copyright 1986, American Medical Association. Reprinted by permission of *JAMA* and the author.

Charts on pages 264 and 268 and the photograph in the insert of an ultrasound recording of fetal heart beats. Reproduced by permission of International Biomedics, Bothell, WA.

Photograph in the insert of a fetus's facial profile. Reproduced by permission of J. Gerald Quirk, Jr., M.D., Ph.D.

All other photographs in the insert reproduced by permission of H. Howard Cockrill, Jr., M.D., and Arkansas Radiology Associates, P.A.

PRIMELIFE PREGNANCY. Copyright © 1987 by Clark Gillespie, M.D. All rights reserved. Printed in the United States of America. No part of this book may be used or reproduced in any manner whatsoever without written permission except in the case of brief quotations embodied in critical articles and reviews. For information address Harper & Row, Publishers, Inc., 10 East 53rd Street, New York, N.Y. 10022. Published simultaneously in Canada by Fitzhenry & Whiteside Limited, Toronto.

FIRST EDITION

*Designed by Ruth Bornschlegel*

Library of Congress Cataloging-in-Publication Data

Gillespie, Clark.
  Primelife pregnancy.

  Includes index.
  1. Pregnancy in middle age.   I. Title.
[DNLM: 1. Maternal Age—popular works.
2. Pregnancy—popular works.   WQ 150 G478p]
RG556.6.G55   1987      618.2′00880565       87–45049
ISBN 0–06–055088–0          87 88 89 90 91 MPC 10 9 8 7 6 5 4 3 2 1
ISBN 0–06–096207–0 (pbk) 87 88 89 90 91 MPC 10 9 8 7 6 5 4 3 2 1

*Dedicated with love to*
*Jann, Cindy, Tiffani, Amanda, and Laura*

# Acknowledgments

The author gratefully acknowledges significant help from the Little Rock Radiology Clinic and in particular from Harry Howard Cockrill, Jr., M.D., from the Department of Obstetrics and Gynecology, The University of Arkansas School of Medicine, and from James Gerald Quirk, M.D.

Also gratefully acknowledged is Lisa Bridges, who graciously typed and retyped the manuscript while committing a number of new expletives to memory—all of which, I hope, have been deleted from the book.

And, finally, Susan, my adorable and forbearing wife, who left me alone when I needed to be left alone and succored me when I needed succoring— what words are good enough?

# Contents

A section of photographs follows page 118.

# ○ Introduction ○

# Follow the Yellow Brick Road

It is clear that more and more women now become pregnant after thirty-five, many for the first time. Goals have contributed heavily to this late surge, but there are many other reasons. To be sure, we all begin to think of our lives in the future when we reach the mid-thirties, but a woman reflects not only on her primal maternal urge and capacity, but also upon the fulfillment of what she perceives to be her life role. As often as not this goal is motherhood. And that leads to the Yellow Brick Road.

The pregnant journey thus about to be encountered is filled with a variety of obstacles, some easy to overstep, some requiring help from others, and some that remain to be dealt with throughout the whole journey. One of the persistent obstacles is age.

Age is not everything. Sometimes we wish it were nothing. Lots of times. But it is there, and we are reminded of it constantly by an age-conscious society. After all, we go to school, can drive, drink, gain our freedom, get drafted, promoted, retired, and finally get social security (if there is any left) all at a certain age. It doesn't always make sense but there it is. And if we happen to forget our age for a moment there are clocks, calendars, an advertising industry, and mirrors all ready to fetch us back on line.

And so we must address pregnancy and age—another time lapse conflict. Having a baby is traditionally a proper event between eighteen and thirty-five. Before eighteen, unless the mother is eating properly, both the mother and baby can suffer. Now, then, after thirty-five—well, after thirty-five women are supposed to have passed instantaneously some biological millennium so that pregnancy becomes an incredible disaster. But does it?

Does the goddess of reproductive health pull up stakes when the clock strikes midnight on your last day of thirty-four? Why not thirty-three or thirty-seven? Who decreed thirty-five?

Here perhaps may be a timely answer. At thirty, a woman's reproductive quality is about as good as it ever can be. At forty, however, both maternal and fetal pregnancy outcome are in significantly greater jeopardy. From thirty upward to forty, the line of obstetrical complications rises slowly at first, then much more rapidly as thirty-five approaches forty—but it is a line not a wall until forty-five.

Doctors and others who devote their lifework to maternal and fetal health needed a reference point to frame the reproductive problems of women in their thirties and that point had to be standardized so that results from around the world are comparable and meaningful to all investigators. Finally, a point needed to be established so that we working obstetricians could change our management protocols and plans, gearing them to the potentially higher risks involved as mothers aged. That selected point, in all cases, is thirty-five.

So, there you have it. In concrete.

But at this juncture it is important to remember that your life and physiology didn't change abruptly the evening before you became thirty-five. It is equally important to remember that changes—many of them subtle—have been going on in your body for some time, even in the most disciplined and healthy body. These changes make certain physiological goals more difficult to achieve. Ask any athlete—it is a fact of life. So there is no question that in later reproductive years, pregnancy is harder to acquire, maintain, and complete successfully. And all this is not alone due to the aging process. Coexisting diseases plus fixed and prolonged bad habits take their toll as well.

On the other side of the coin, *you* have developed values, stability, and self-control in mastering your goals—all valuable tools for what you have now undertaken. Moreover, you are more likely to comply with what you are asked to do and with advice and information that you perceive to be correct. Further, with the surge of interest in healthy bodies, your self-care has probably taken a significant turn for the better and you are more likely treating your body like a temple rather than an ashtray—or a septic tank. And finally, modern reproductive technology is pushing aside many of the problems associated with a mature ("age" will *not* again be mentioned in this book) pregnancy and almost all of these newer techniques are available anywhere in this country.

Some women now experiencing a primelife pregnancy have delivered in the past before entering the sacrosanct "over thirty-five" dominion. Their pregnancies and deliveries may very well have been quite normal and without any difficulties. If so, this may make the extra attention now required by their present pregnancies seem to them superfluous and contrived.

Not so.

Clearly, a pregnancy carried to fruition by a mother over thirty-five is a special situation requiring special attention—regardless of all previous reproductive experience, good or bad. The special circumstances may be explained by comparing a lazy afternoon drive in clear weather to flying the same route by instruments through a thunderstorm. Both have inherent problems and risks but the flight—like the primelife pregnancy—requires more skills and intensive monitoring. With care both conclude safely.

So even as late as forty-five, if you move out of the fast lane, bond with a reasonable and caring obstetrician, manage your equipment well, accept some technical procedures as necessary and protective, then you are likely to achieve your primelife obstetrical goal with safety and success.

What follows are the facts of life, pregnancy, and birth in such a mature environment.

The first five chapters of this book are made up of advice, information, and instructions related to your pregnancy and to be modified by your personal physician and your own wisdom, and not to be taken as marble brought down by Moses. Many variations of good and standard care exist here and elsewhere and there are geographical, physical, climatalogical, cultural, social, and financial variables which alter circumstances. Your own physician is your best adviser.

The next two chapters deal with problems that may arise in primelife pregnancies and with already existing problems and how generally they are dealt with. The final two chapters detail the technology referred to in the earlier chapters.

Because we live in a world where social values are in a state of rapid flux and, for good or for bad, most of the social mores and folkways with which we grew up do not exist anymore, it is no longer possible to write a pregnancy self-help book and identify your unimpregnated coconspirator as your husband. Indeed, that may be your situation but statistics increasingly argue against it. Regardless, we have happily removed two words from our book's lexicon—*age* and *fat*—and reluctantly remove one other, *husband.*

# PART 1

# YOUR PREGNANCY

This book is made up of advice, information, and instructions related to your pregnancy and to be modified by your personal physician and your own wisdom. Many variations of good and standard care exist here and elsewhere and there are geographic, physical, climatological, cultural, social, and financial variables that alter circumstances. Your own physician is your best adviser.

○ ] ○

# Early Pregnancy

## HOW PREGNANCY OCCURS

That's probably the funniest line you will read in this book. Every child in every household with cable TV already knows as much as we do about *how*. Granted, the opportunity and experience doesn't exist as frequently as the tube leads them to believe, but all else is factual. Those who miss the TV learning experience can pick it up at a friendly newsstand or at the next bunking party. So what I have to say is brief—just the skimpy facts.

If all goes well during the warm, interpersonal relationship of lovemaking, millions of sperm are deposited in the back of the vagina during male orgasm. Many migrate up the uterine opening (cervix) and through the uterus into the tubes. If the customary midmonth ovulation has taken place, a receptive egg is in one of these tubes and one sperm of the advancing horde gets to do the honors and so fertilization occurs as the sperm unites with the egg. Over the next several days, the budding embryo moves down the tube and into the uterus where it embeds for some 260 days or so.

Two hormone events happen at this time and are important to record. First, the ovary at the site of ovulation forms a cyst (corpus luteum) which produces progesterone—a hormone and an immunosuppressant—which helps prevent rejection of the fetus—a foreign graft. Eventually, progesterone secretions are taken over by the placenta.

The other hormone made entirely by what will become the placenta—chorionic embryo tissue—is called chorionic gonado-tropin (CGT) or human chorionic gonadotropin (HCG), the more common designation. This is a multipurpose hormone and we use it to detect pregnancy and to monitor its health in early months.

And that's about all there is to it. Stripped of the social, moral, legal, ethical, financial, and sensual side issues, it is a pretty straightforward affair. The whole process will be described in more detail in the later chapters in this book, but for now, that's enough. Let's move on.

## DIAGNOSIS OF PREGNANCY

### By personal signs and symptoms

○ Missed period. There are many things that interfere with normal menses—stress, illness, exercise, etc.—but a missed period is commonly the first indication of a pregnancy and should be so regarded.

○ Engorged and tender breasts. Breast discomfort is generally greater than is usually felt just before a normal period. You feel like you want to carry your breasts in a box—a mummy box, not a jewel box.

○ Digestive insults. Nausea—even vomiting—is not uncommon. The smoke-filled room—which you should avoid anyway—will make you gag. Things you liked—people's cooking you once liked, even your own cooking—may repeal your own sensitive stomach.

○ Fatigue. If you thought you were tired after your first weekend encounter session or after you had your mother underfoot for a week, you haven't really tasted exhaustion. You will know it soon.

○ Frequency. Because of local congestion, the bladder feels put upon and asks to be emptied much more—night and day.

○ Emotions. Although the pregnancy has been planned and wished for, depression and irritability with many episodes of unexplainable tears may befall you—for a while.

## By examination

It is difficult for a physician to diagnosis pregnancy before the second missed period. Most of the early diagnostic signs are due to breast and uterine congestion.

○ Breasts. Human chorionic gonadotropin (HCG) causes intense reaction and swelling in breast tissues. On examination the breasts are very firm and tender and the veins just under the skin become dilated and easily visible. Often a clear secretion can be expressed from the nipples. Called colostrum, it is the forerunner of milk. This sign is only of value in the first pregnancy because once one pregnancy, always breast secretions.

○ HCG also produces marked swelling in the uterus and surrounding tissues. The cervix appears blue and feels softened. The uterine body also feels softer and more globular. Rarely, the normal cyst of pregnancy can be felt on the ovary from which the now fertile egg originally ruptured. This, however, is not a dependable sign.

## By pregnancy testing

Many reliable types of pregnancy tests now exist for use both at home and in the laboratory. Although they vary in procedure, they are nevertheless all based upon reactions to human chorionic gonadotropin (HCG). You remember that the budding placenta produces this hormone within a few days after fertilization. HCG is circulated in the blood and excreted and concentrated in the urine—the more concentrated the urine, the more accurate the test. That's why early morning specimens are more sensitive. Blood specimens are as good one time as another since the blood concentration of HCG does not normally vary.

○ Urine pregnancy test kits contain red blood cells which have been coated with HCG antigen in the laboratory. The kits also contain an HCG antibody. When the two are mixed together they clump—and you can see it. However, if you add urine to the mixture and that urine contains HCG, the clumping is prevented because the HCG antibody is neutralized by the HCG in the urine. Thus, no clumps means the test is positive, and it's time to reach for the phone.

o Blood pregnancy tests are more sensitive and more accurate. Involved here is a radioimmunoassay technique which earned a Nobel prize for the discoverer. Such tests are dependable seven to ten days after a missed period.

o The most accurate pregnancy test available for clinical use today is the beta HCG determination. Beta HCG is a small, very specific fraction of the whole HCG spectrum. Modern testing can measure as few as five and as many as 100,000 units of beta HCG in the blood. Thus, pregnancy can be detected before a missed period and the health of a pregnancy—even its location—can be followed. More of this later.

## By ultrasound

This modern laboratory tool has indeed revolutionized pregnancy management, and is involved in studying all stages of pregnancy in a variety of ways. In the beginning, ultrasound can detect, with accuracy and safety, the location, duration, and health of any pregnancy. Such information derived without risk is often of incredible help. A fetal sac with a fetal pole can be visualized when the pregnancy has existed about one month and the fetal heart can be seen beating shortly thereafter. Truly remarkable!

To sum up, there are many ways to determine the presence of pregnancy both early and accurately—and all of them are safe. Some are expensive—but again they are all safe. Your biggest problem is going to be who to tell first. That used to be your husband, but with today's life-style, your mate has already figured it out. The problem comes in telling your employer, employees, associates, customers, and clients.

Once pregnancy has been established and all "need to know" parties know, and the maternity backlash from nonpregnant women in your occupational community has been resolved or temporized, here is a list of probable dos and don'ts that you might contemplate:

**DO**

- Get an obstetrician if you do not already have one. See below.
- Eat well. If you are nauseated, see pages 24–25.
- Share a sip of champagne. Share most of it since you need to restrict alcohol. See pages 64–65.
- Spread the news among those who don't need to know.
- Make love—tenderly.

**DON'T**

- Diet in any way or try to lose weight.
- Take drugs or medications of *any* kind.
- Smoke or allow anyone to smoke around you, at home or at work.
- Drink alcohol—except for the exception above.
- Expose yourself to toxic substances in the work place or at home. This involves many types of pollutants— even some hobbies and some common household chemicals. See pages 19 and 41–42.
- Travel. In the early months stay close to your base, and avoid significant altitude changes. See pages 82–85.
- Overdo physical activity. Exercise is great but in reasonable doses. See pages 34–41.
- Handle pets. See pages 42–45.

## FINDING A DOCTOR

A primelife pregnancy deserves the extra care that a qualified obstetrician can provide. In some situations—particularly if there are preexisting maternal health problems or a previous complicated pregnancy—the help of a perinatologist may be required. This particular obstetrician has had special training and certification in maternal-fetal medicine and is only available at level III maternity centers. (See pages 240–41.) Generally, though, a regular obstetrician fills the bill and they practice in most areas of our country. Sad to say, they are becoming scarce in some high density states on the east and west coasts. Malpractice costs and risks are forcing them to give up their lifework. In some parts of New York State, for instance, malpractice premiums cost $80,000 each year, and some are expected to reach $100,000! This is too much to absorb and too much to pass on to patients—who are the ultimate funders of the malpractice lottery.

You will certainly want an obstetrician who is in agreement with your goals. Decide if you want a physician who practices alone or is one in a group. He or she must practice alone *if* you prefer to have one person to relate to in this very personal area. But remember, doctors have to be away sometimes and so a stranger may be answering your calls at times. On the other hand, your doctor must practice in a group if you want to be certain that a physician with your records is always available. It's harder to bond to a group, but doctor bonding may not be as important to you as it was to other generations.

Be sure your doctors use the hospital of your choice—or that their hospital fills equally well your needs for a particular birth environment. Maternity hospitals are glad to share this information with prospective mothers.

Find out if your doctors are involved with the type of birth program that meets your wishes. That would involve areas like preparation classes, birth suites, sibling programs, as well as pain relief programs. This information is generally made available by the doctors' staff and there is no need to confront the doctors to learn their positions. Hospitals and other patients will also be information sources.

Check credentials. Obstetricians are certified by the American Board of Obstetricians and Gynecologists and each has a diploma to that effect. They *all* must now recertify every ten years. In addition, most belong to the American College of Obstetricians and Gynecologists. The college, too, demands a certifying examination. Most obstetricians belong to both organizations—all of them to at least one. Finally, many private obstetricians have teaching appointments if there is a local medical school. This helps the doctor keep current and helps medical students understand private patient problems and viewpoints.

## MEETING HIM/HER/THEM

Your primelife pregnancy is important to you and you want to document it early and determine its well-being so visit your obstetrician early. Pregnancy, as you are now aware, can be diagnosed early, and in case you anticipate any problems, it is well to have adequate early records. *Accurate* dating of the pregnancy and the measured health of that pregnancy are often important. Such parameters are now readily available.

### First visit—what happens?

° You give a complete history of your medical and social background. This history may be taken by the obstetrician, by an associate, or it may be a checklist that you fill out yourself. Some things that you are asked to record do not seem important, but they generally are. You will see this for yourself as our handbook unfolds.

° You have a general physical as well as pelvic examination as the next step. Special attention is drawn to any preexisting medical problems you may have.

° Laboratory tests are done. If due, a Pap smear is taken during the pelvic examination. Sometimes a vaginal culture is also taken at that time. If there is any question about the duration or health of the pregnancy, an ultrasound scan may be done. Some doctors refer these examinations to radiology clinics and so the procedure may be deferred a few days. Blood is drawn and submitted for routine counting plus tests for syphilis (the law), for certain antibodies, particularly rubella (German measles), toxoplasmosis (cat fever, see page 125), for blood typing, and Rh factor, and anything else appropriate for your personal care. A regular and routine urinalysis is also done.

Other special tests may be indicated. For example, if there is a history of breast cancer on the maternal side of your family—and particularly if the onset was early in occurring—you may have a mammogram (breast x-ray). Not to worry—you will be adequately screened to protect your pregnancy from the *minimal* x-ray exposure involved. Another example: If, say, you are diabetic, then special blood studies may be conducted to assess your current status. And so on. These special laboratory studies for special conditions are generally covered in the second section of this book as these conditions unfold.

○ Finally, when all this is over, you have a conference with your doctor to see if you have passed or failed and you get your instructions and vitamin/mineral supplements. Listen to your doctor. As I have already said, you are much more likely to listen than the average new mother. But hear this. It doesn't matter whether you consider your doctors as paid providers, whether you hang on every word they utter, or whatever—compliance is important. Not for better marks or a smoother, less confrontational relationship. But for the attainment of your goal—pure and simple—compliance is important and its importance is demonstrated over and over as we move along.

○ Your discussion with each other centers on routine care, and also upon special procedures related to the health of a primelife pregnancy. You will hear about some things already familiar to you and about certain new ones. Thus, *amniocentesis* is bandied about as well as *biophysical profiles, stress testing,* and more. Further, if you have a specific medical problem (diabetes, hypertension, or obesity, for example) special advice is given in those areas.

## SUBSEQUENT VISITS

Visits to the obstetrician increase in frequency as the pregnancy approaches maturity. Most often a monthly checkup suffices at first and the gap gradually closes so that at full term once a week is the rule. This is not always the case, however. There are certain pregnancy situations which, in any age bracket, call for more frequent visits. As an example, if high blood pressure appears at any time, it is wise not to neglect such a finding and more frequent examinations are necessary to determine the hypertension's course, its possible effect on both mother and baby, and the results of treatment. At times this may require almost daily visits. Associated health hazards such as diabetes, chronic preexisting hypertension, etc., also demand a schedule of encounters that are best mapped out individually—and may be at great variance with what is held to be routine.

What happens at a routine return visit? Almost always you will be flat on your back when you see your doctor for return appointments. This is a very bad bargaining position and, to say the least, not an elegant way to carry out any social, nonsexual encounter of which I am aware. This unsuitable arrangement is gradually yielding with better exam room equipment and more sensitive physicians. For the moment at hand, you have been weighed already, your blood pressure has been taken, and a urine specimen evaluated. The big number comes in, asks a cluster of relevant questions which may not seem to be relevant questions, feels your abdomen, listens for a fetal heart with a monitor that lets you hear too—hopefully—and, unless you have a problem area that needs attention (vaginal discharge, for instance), that's about it. Eventually you are sitting up and able to have a direct eyeball-to-eyeball discussion of any problems you have. Remember, this is a routine examination and just the framework on which your pregnancy development hangs. Many other things are added as you already know and will learn of as we move on.

## VISITATION ETIQUETTE

This is a two-edged sword. Certain demands are put upon both you and the doctor to make your regular conferences a meeting of the minds rather than a series of confrontations—like a visit with your parole officer.

Have a ready list of things about which you need to ask. You can use areas of my book to list your questions or you may use any reliable recording source.

Don't be afraid to be a little dependent. You have consciously selected your doctor and that is a very important talisman in the developing relationship between the two of you. Regardless of the current move to reduce a doctor-patient relationship to a client-provider relationship, and regardless of the altruistic intent behind such a drive, it simply won't wash in the long run. And there is no reason why it should—there is absolutely nothing to be gained and much to be lost by such a resolution of meaningful interpersonal contact. The doctor-patient relationship is a dependent one. Granted. But so is the pilot-passenger relationship. And I, for one, cherish that relationship. There is nothing wrong with a limited short-term dependency, and in the long run, much to be gained. Human frailty is what it is and exists everywhere but trust you must to survive. And who better to trust and to lay a little dependency on—outside the framework of your own loved one—than the person who is ultimately responsible for the safe deliverance of you and your babe? So, open up a bit.

## THE TELEPHONE

Since the United States government in its infinite wisdom decided we no longer need good telephone service, you may or may not be able to communicate directly at all times with your doctor anymore. Even in the unusual event that the phones do work well, there is still often a medical answering service standing between the two of you particularly when your need appears greatest—nights and weekends. But remember, such services are paid to seek and find—not lose and hide your doctor. So don't take any lip from them. When you do get to talk to the doctor, remember the rules of the ring:

   ○ Don't call unless it's basic and urgent. Write down routine questions in your handbook so that you can ask them at the office and not on the phone. The doctor is less rushed and busy at nights and on weekends, and really wants it that way. That's fair enough.

   ○ Give your name and the duration of your pregnancy. Your obstetrician knows you—knows and remembers all about you and your pregnancy—and 300 others—but it is a nice little touch that you can add to sort of personalize things. After all, you do that much when you call the vet about your puppy.

   ○ Don't—repeat—*don't* have anyone call for you if you can possibly call yourself. This avoids secondhand information or a shouting match, or both, neither of which leads to wisdom—or problem solving.

   ○ Have the phone number of your druggist close by in the unlikely event that the doctor orders something helpful for you. There is little helpful medication left that we can order.

○ Many times trained office personnel—particularly nurse practitioners—can answer your questions. These assistants are pretty well aware of their limitations and their liabilities in today's world, so they are not likely to accept responsibilities that exceed their ability to solve. You can generally go with their advice.

## THE WORK PLACE: FOR WHOM THE BELLE TOILS

Not so long ago, being pregnant and gainfully employed outside the home presented no problem whatsoever. As soon as the pregnancy declared itself, the bearer was fired—perhaps to be rehired sometime in the future, perhaps not. After all, America is—or was—a work ethic society and business is business. So that was it.

This state of affairs existed until quite recently in our work environment. Business attitudes began to change as more and more women entered the work force and as some women began challenging their employer's pregnancy policies in court. These actions resulted largely in favorable decisions for working pregnant women. But there is still a long way to go. Most authoritative help comes from OSHA (Occupational Safety and Health Administration), and through the Pregnancy Discrimination Act passed in 1979 as an amendment to the Civil Rights Act of 1964. Even so, only 40 percent of employed American women are entitled to six weeks' paid pregnancy leave! Records obtained from *over 100 other countries* reveal that most mature societies allow pregnant women leave with no loss of benefits for up to nine months! In some countries (Sweden, for instance), pay as well as benefits continue throughout that leave. The current attitude of business in America, then, toward pregnancy in the work force is somewhat equivalent to that of an emerging Third World nation.

Regardless of all this, we have to address certain real problems that exist in deciding work guidelines for pregnant women. These include your wishes, your health, the type of work you do (sedentary, physical, hazardous, toxic exposure, etc.), and company policy and legal liability. Employers do not like to be sued for dismissing or, on the other hand, endangering their pregnant employees.

Let us summarize these points.

## Your wishes

Many goal-oriented pregnant women want to work as long as they can and return very quickly. In many cases there is considerable pressure exerted upon them to stay late and return early. This pressure, interestingly, often arises from other female employees who do not want their employer to have any case examples of pregnancy interfering with work responsibilities—examples that can be used in future negotiations against advancement and increased responsibilities. A strange twist!

On the other side of the coin, some pregnant workers, even though healthy and in sedentary work, may want extensive leave before and/or after delivery. These situations require negotiation.

## Your health

Certain pregnant patients have complicating medical problems that warrant restrictions in work duration. Examples include:

○ Previous delivery of two premature infants, whether it be due to a weakened cervix, congenital abnormalities of the uterus, or other unknown causes.

○ Significant heart disease.

○ Significant high blood pressure.

○ Certain diabetics.

○ Severe anemias and certain other blood disorders.

○ Systemic diseases, such as kidney disease, convulsive states, crippling orthopedic limitations, and so on.

○ There are also, of course, a number of pure obstetrical complications that either terminate work at once or modify its continuation. These include such events as vaginal bleeding, ruptured membranes, abnormal placental location, and multiple infants. There are others, and your obstetrician will be your guide.

# The type of work you do

The list on page 20 is relatively complete, but is constantly changing, and again, your own obstetrician is your best and final guide. All of it, of course, relates to the physical level of the occupation.

Any occupation that embraces hazardous and toxic material should be avoided. Here is a list of most known toxins that may be present in certain work environments:*

○ Heavy metals—cadmium, lead, and mercury.

○ Solvents—benzene.

○ Halogenated hydrocarbons—chloropreme, dichloro-bromopropane, epichlorohydrin, ethylene dibromide, polychlorinated biphenyls (PCBs), tetrachlorethylene, vinyl chloride, ethyleneglycol, ethylene oxide, formaldehyde. All of the above groups may be found in a variety of industrial sources.

○ Anesthetic gases—all halogenated gases—e.g., methoxyflurane.

○ Pesticides—carbaryl, chlordane and kepone, DDT, endrin, lindane, and others.

○ DES—an estrogenlike compound used in feeding and fattening some animals for slaughter.

○ Radiation. Unless closely monitored, work in hospitals, clinics, dental offices, and certain industries may expose employees to significant radiation. Incidentally, no significant data has accumulated at this writing to prove that computer terminals pose a radiation risk to pregnant or nonpregnant workers.

Certain other work environments may pose specific hazards to pregnancy. These include:

○ Exposure to dangerous bacteria and viruses—e.g., oral surgery and dialysis units (hepatitis, AIDS?), pet shops (toxoplasmosis), teaching (rubella).

---

*Source: American College of Obstetricians and Gynecologists, *Guidelines on Pregnancy and Work,* p. 16. Washington, D.C.: ACOG, 1977.

## WHAT RESTRICTIONS DO PHYSICIANS SUGGEST FOR WORKING PATIENTS WITH NORMAL PREGNANCIES?

This summary of *Contemporary Ob/Gyn* survey results shows that the advice readers give is closely related to job demands. Here the "All Jobs" section indicates suggestions for sedentary workers that apply equally to those engaged in more energetic activities.

---

### ALL JOBS

TRY TO:

Take frequent breaks
Rest on left side at lunch hour
Stop working when fatigued
Elevate legs periodically
Take walks
Perform stretching exercises, especially for back and legs
Wear support hose

AVOID:

Exhaustion
Discomfort
Strenuous exercise
Extreme temperatures
Smoking areas
Noxious odors and chemical fumes
Ladder climbing
Lifting more than 10, 15, or 25 pounds [different responses]

---

### JOBS THAT REQUIRE STANDING OR WALKING

TRY TO:

Reduce activity; work part-time or at most in 8-hour shifts
Take naps or rest periods morning and afternoon
Empty bladder every 2 hours
Stop or reduce work 2 to 4 weeks before EDC

AVOID:

Heavy lifting or pushing
Excessive stair climbing
Running
In-flight airline work in final month

---

### JOBS THAT REQUIRE PHYSICAL EXERTION

TRY TO:

Use common sense
Stop when short of breath
Sleep on left side
Empty bladder every 2 hours
Get extra rest on weekends
Exercise great caution around hazardous equipment, such as machinery with moving parts
Stop work after 7 to 8 months' gestation
Work part-time (20 hours per week) for 2 to 4 weeks before EDC

AVOID:

Heavy lifting and straining
Jogging and contact sports
Prolonged standing or walking
Horseback riding, skiing, rough hiking after 7 months
Trauma to abdomen from heavy equipment
Overtime

Source: *Contemporary Ob/Gyn,* Medical Economics Company.

o Work that is excessively physical, involves long hours and high stress.

o Work that involves continued physical dexterity and motion.

o Very recently American Telephone and Telegraph (AT&T) banned pregnant women from its semiconductor production lines, citing a Massachusetts health study report that showed an increased miscarriage rate in female assembly-line workers. An assortment of toxic gases and chemicals is involved in chip etching. Other Silicon Valley chip makers may soon follow suit. AT&T offers transfer of pregnant women to other job responsibilities.

## Company policy

Most companies have pregnancy employment guidelines which take the above material into account and most companies do their best to protect their pregnant employees. Sometimes your obstetrician needs to help your employer apply these guidelines and most of us are very willing to do so. The employer has many things to consider, not the least of which is his legal liability at *both* ends of the stick. Policies are becoming more liberal and protective but we still have a ways to go.

Remember one thing clearly—the guidelines on page 22 will change as time goes on, and your obstetrician is more current than any book can be.

It should be noted that the United States Supreme Court recently ruled that states may enact laws requiring employers to provide unpaid leave and reinstatement to pregnant women. They ruled favorably on such a law passed in California. At least eight additional states—Connecticut, Hawaii, Illinois, Massachusetts, Montana, New Hampshire, Ohio, and Washington—have similar laws. There is now an act before Congress introduced in April 1985 by Representative Patricia Schroeder (D-Colorado) which requires all employers to provide a minimum of eighteen weeks' unpaid leave for any employee who chooses to stay home to care for a newborn, newly adopted, or seriously ill child. The employee must be reinstated to the same job at the same pay upon return. It also requires the employer to maintain the employee's health insurance benefits through the leave period.

# HOW LONG MAY WOMEN WORK? GENERAL GUIDELINES FROM THE AMERICAN MEDICAL ASSOCIATION

WEEK OF GESTATION

FIRST TRIMESTER: 1 2 3 4 5 6 7 8 9 10 11 12 — SECOND TRIMESTER: 13 14 15 16 17 18 19 20 21 22 23 24 25 26 27 28 29 — THIRD TRIMESTER: 30 31 32 33 34 35 36 37 38 39 40

| JOB FUNCTION | May work until week |
|---|---|
| SECRETARIAL, LIGHT CLERICAL, PROFESSIONAL, MANAGERIAL | 40 |
| SEATED, LIGHT TASKS (prolonged or intermittent) | 40 |
| STANDING — Prolonged (>4 hrs) | 24 |
| STANDING — Intermittent (>30 mins/hr) | 32 |
| STANDING — (<30 mins/hr) | 40 |
| STOOPING AND BENDING BELOW KNEE LEVEL — Repetitive (>10 times/hr) | 20 |
| STOOPING AND BENDING BELOW KNEE LEVEL — Intermittent (<10 >2 times/hr) | 28 |
| STOOPING AND BENDING BELOW KNEE LEVEL — (<2 times/hr) | 40 |
| CLIMBING LADDERS AND POLES — Repetitive (>4 times/8-hr shift) | 20 |
| CLIMBING LADDERS AND POLES — Intermittent (<4 times/8-hr shift) | 28 |
| CLIMBING STAIRS — Repetitive (>4 times/8-hr shift) | 28 |
| CLIMBING STAIRS — Intermittent (<4 times/8-hr shift) | 40 |
| LIFTING, REPETITIVE — >50 lbs | 20 |
| LIFTING, REPETITIVE — <50 >25 lbs | 24 |
| LIFTING, REPETITIVE — <25 lbs | 40 |
| LIFTING, INTERMITTENT — >50 lbs | 30 |
| LIFTING, INTERMITTENT — <50 >25 lbs | 40 |
| LIFTING, INTERMITTENT — >25 lbs | 40 |

Source: Contemporary Ob/Gyn, Medical Economics Company.

Called the Parental and Disability Leave Act of 1985 (H.R. 2020), it contains other provisions to raise the disability and parental leave benefits to the level of other industrialized nations, in which regard, we, the United States, are dead last.

## SOME MORE THOUGHT ABOUT WORK

A recent survey revealed that major corporations displayed very variable maternity leave policies. Two thirds allowed up to eight weeks' leave. A small number allowed as much as twelve weeks, while another fraction felt that one to four weeks was enough. About 40 percent offered unpaid paternity and adoptive parent leave.

Although children raised in working mother households seem to develop and thrive as well as any other child, going back to work—and the timing of it—often presents a crisis to the mother. Here are some ideas:

○ Get as much maternity leave as you can—consistent with your own career goals and what your company will offer. H.R. 2020 should soon become law.

○ Part-time, compressed-time, or job-sharing relationships may work for you. Moreover, it is becoming increasingly popular to allow computer-linked work to be done at home. And everything but the company restrooms seem to be computer-linked today.

○ Paternity leave is becoming more common and more acceptable at corporate levels. Some men just take off a year (Ted Koppel is one of them, but there are plenty of others) to share this deeply involved aspect of parenting.

○ If your unimpregnanted coconspirator cannot get away from his work, he must still be there as much as possible to be supportive of you and the little one. Being supportive often means emotional guidance, physical and financial protection, and masculine role playing. It also means night work, diaper changing, cooking, dishwashing, and general scut work.

○ Try and resolve your conflicts about work and what it means to your relationship with your child before you return to work. Get your priorities listed and in order. Carry them to work with you instead of guilt.

## SOME EARLY NUISANCES

Early on I mentioned some of the opening symptoms of pregnancy. They can really be a nuisance, particularly if you are working or if you have small children, so here is a little more information about them:

### Nausea and vomiting

You have become the host to your soon-to-be infant and as such you have accepted a foreign tissue graft to your body—an allograft is what the little troublemaker is called. No matter what it is called, your immune system has to be brought to its knees or else you will abort—just like people reject other organ transplants unless their rejection mechanisms are suppressed. In order to do this, you, at first, and then the placenta secrete the necessary substances and in the beginning these substances may nauseate you. And there you have it, pure and simple. The first thing that *you* will notice is that you can smell an egg through its shell.

The nausea is usually most bothersome when your stomach is most empty (the mornings), or the most irritated (pizza, taco, barbecue), or the most stuffed (whenever you can get to do it). So here are some hints:

○ Eat in small amounts and frequently. Eat a little before bed, again if you are up at night tending to other problems, and in the morning as soon as you awaken. Then nibble during the day but with no set *big* mealtimes.

○ Avoid seasoned, greasy, or rich foods. Try and choose from the diet outline on page 50. But whatever you do, break up your meals into little snacks.

○ When you get feeling good again, don't go for broke. No feasts or food orgies just yet.

○ If your vitamin/mineral preparation nauseates you, particularly if you regurgitate it, take it with some food, or if you must, leave it off for a week and try again.

○ Do not take medications, however safe, for nausea. You can use vitamin B6 tablets—100 mg three times daily—for some relief if your own doctor agrees.

○ If you smoke—which you shouldn't—don't. Avoid smoke-filled rooms or odorous rooms of any kind. Your employer *must* provide you with a smoke-free environment.

Sometimes—but rarely—severe nausea and vomiting can lead to dehydration and require temporary hospitalization. Call your doctor if your mouth and your skin are dry, if nothing stays down and you are losing weight. Incidentally, repeated vomiting may be accompanied by some fine strings of blood-tinged mucous. This is from the stomach irritation and is not serious unless persistent.

Generally your body adjusts by the third month and the nausea abates—and there is a world of sinful things out there waiting for you. If you are a lawyer, a torte takes on a sinful new meaning; if you are a hunter, mousse is a brand-new game; and if you are into stocks and bonds, the market is now at your delicatessen. More on that later.

## Fatigue

Your body has now been put to work on triple shifts and it soon shows. The six o'clock news signals bedtime and the weekends fade into dreamland. Not only has your energy deserted you but you tend to get dizzy easily and may fold from the scene completely if wherever you happen to be is too hot or too crowded—and if you bound out of bed in the morning, they may find you hooked on the bathroom door. And so on. You are not exactly your old electric self, and you are only a nighttime person when it comes to bladder function. This too shall pass but until it does, you had best give in to it.

○ Go to bed early—listen to your body signals.

○ Don't get up quickly and avoid standing for long periods of time without moving around. If you are of Episcopal or Catholic faith, don't stay on your knees too long.

○ Avoid crowded, congested hot or humid areas. I suppose that includes most urban areas today.

° If you feel faint—no matter where you are—get down and stay down, sitting or resting on your side till help comes and the feeling passes. Be careful the remainder of the day.

## Tenderness

° Breasts. The full, congested feeling you have experienced will leave in a few weeks. Until it does don't do anything that makes your breasts move faster than you do, and don't hug anybody. No matter what is in vogue at this time, wear some support—even in bed—till comfort returns. Your breasts will soon begin to secrete a clear liquid (colostrum) off and on throughout pregnancy and it can stain your clothing. The secretion is slightly bitter and often flows freely during foreplay. Just an observation for you to file away. You will also notice more breast secretions if you jog.

Your breasts will most likely increase somewhat in size during pregnancy and your cup may increase in size—and length. More about this and other breast matters later.

° Emotions. This is a time for tenderness. The emotions for many reasons become somewhat brittle even if all things are as they should be. You may slip into a minor tearful depressive episode for no apparent cause that vanishes as quickly as it came. There usually won't be a reason. Tenderness is what helps. And closeness. These episodes generally leave early on—sometimes to return for a few days after delivery, sometimes never to return.

## DISCOMFORT

In a healthy primelife pregnancy, some minor but often persistent discomforts mar an otherwise delightful experience. Nausea, breast tenderness, fatigue, and emotional lumps have already been laid before you. But there is more.

Lower abdominal discomfort may arise from several benign sources. Remember, lower abdominal pain and cramping, particularly if accompanied by bleeding, *may* signal a threatened abortion or, worse, an ectopic pregnancy. Don't neglect these signs. But here are some other sources of pain that will, of their own, pass into oblivion:

○ Uterine cramps. Your baby, as you are now aware, is a graft—partly yours, partly someone else's. Your uterus has to accept this graft and grow with it. Sometimes the uterus fights back and so cramping occurs. Usually it is light. It may be more evident when you are missing a period, but this is not always so. When it happens, slow down and lay back. Should the cramping become regular and painful or should any vaginal blood appear, report. Something else is going on. The nonsignificant type of cramping generally disappears by the fourth month.

○ Ligament pain. As your uterus grows it puts tension on its supporting uterine ligaments. This tension is generally more intense on the right side but not always. The discomfort is felt as a minor pulling-type pain and is accentuated by rapid movement or turning. The whole thing ends after the first few months and is replaced by other character developing situations. It is of no consequence to the pregnancy outcome, but it is another reason to avoid sudden posture changes.

○ Corpus luteum cyst. As you already have learned, a physiological cyst develops on the ovary from which the now fertile egg previously erupted. This cyst makes progesterone, which prevents your cramping uterus from rejecting your little graft. This corpus luteum cyst involutes after the third month, but sometimes can cause some pain on the side on which it resides. Such unilateral cramping may also be an ectopic pregnancy signal, so it should not be ignored. Once you are assured, you may go about your business. Very, very rarely a corpus luteum cyst will rupture, producing severe crippling pain which requires immediate attention. You would know if should it happen, believe me. But it's rare.

## PSEUDOCYESIS

Thoughts and wishes concerning pregnancy awaken many primal urges in a woman's mind. Indeed, the desire to be pregnant may overwhelm the subconscious and, for a fact, set into motion a chain of happenings in the physical body that cannot—at least without study—be distinguished from a true pregnancy. This is pseudocyesis. In such cases, menstruation ceases, breasts grow, get engorged, are tender—even secrete! Fatigue and nausea follow, and in time, abdominal enlargement with striae of pregnancy can occur. These unfortunate women often defer routine obstetrical examinations—which would burst their bubble—and thus sometimes appear at a hospital in labor. So faithfully do their symptoms mimic the real thing that physicians may be drawn into the web of illusion—I have seen residents *follow* and *chart* a case of pseudocyesis through several hours of labor! There are even instances of such bizarre conditions years after a hysterectomy has been performed and pregnancy is no longer possible.

Direct confrontation—even with infallible proof—does not very often suffice to convince a very unhappy pseudomother that she is indeed not pregnant. Even the prolonged passage of time does not blunt their optimism. Professional counseling is the key to their eventual release from this false bondage.

Some men undergo a false pregnancy of sorts while following their mates through the course of pregnancy. Thus, they get up in the morning and throw up as faithfully as she does—and grow a stomach as the months go by. This strange happenstance is called the couvade syndrome. Alas, the male stomach is likely to stay on after the pregnancy is over.

## EARLY PREGNANCY LOSS

This is the time when most spontaneous abortions (miscarriages) take place and also when most ectopic pregnancies will be discovered and removed. Although a great deal more will be said about these two unhappy complications later (pages 206–10), you need to know about them now.

Abortion: There are many conditions which will produce a spontaneous pregnancy loss in the first three or four months and these are listed in the pages noted above. Most often abortion happens because conditions exist which make continued embryo growth and development impossible and your body's protective scanning devices recognize this and so abortion occurs. Sometimes, however, the fetus dies a considerable number of days or even weeks before the abortion takes place and infrequently your doctor, having determined this fact for sure, must initiate the abortion him- or herself. This particular medical grief is called a missed abortion.

The signs and symptoms of abortion include loss of pregnancy feelings (e.g., cessation of nausea) along with some cramping and bleeding. The cramping may be light and the bleeding dark and scanty, but both will increase sooner or later. Rarely do these symptoms mean anything since they can appear in a healthy pregnancy. Nevertheless they should be reported so someone else can make that judgment.

Your doctor's examination may reveal that the uterus is smaller and tender and that the cervix is opening. As further confirmation the beta HCG level will be low and decreasing and an ultrasound examination will generally show an empty fetal sac and that no heartbeat is present.

Most often, once the diagnosis is established, a D & C (dilatation and curettage) will be performed, requiring light anesthesia and a few hours in the hospital. Be sure if you are Rh negative that you get vaccinated (see pages 120–23). You can resume full activity in a few days, but don't get pregnant.

When you have an abortion, particularly if it is your first pregnancy, you will feel the loss, will grieve, and even have some guilt. These are normal responses to a loss of this severity and will leave you when the time is right. Continue to have faith.

The rate of spontaneous abortion is very, very high at any time in life because there is so much that can go wrong. But it is not often a recurrent problem as you can see by reading pages 206–9. Therefore believe because there is more to come. And it's going to be good.

## ECTOPIC PREGNANCY

There are other things that can make you bleed and cramp in early pregnancy. Some of them may be nothing. But one of them could be an ectopic, a pregnancy located outside the uterus, usually in a tube but sometimes in an ovary and even free in the abdomen! That's right. Abdominal ectopic pregnancies have happened—even gone to full term and lived, although they are rare.

So the most common ectopic site is in one tube or the other

where the pregnancy has arrested for some reason and put out its roots. It cannot survive here long because the tube cannot forever expand and it will surely rupture, posing a tremendous surgical emergency.

The usual signs of an ectopic are cramping and light bleeding. The cramping is more likely to be off to one side rather than central as in an abortion, but it is often confusing. You should report the symptoms early on. Generally on examination the doctor can feel the suspicious tubal swelling but it isn't always possible. Thus significant help comes from the lab. Beta HCG levels are generally low and dropping and ultrasound scans show an empty uterus with a fetal sac in the affected tube. Believe me, it's not always that easy.

The treatment is to open the abdomen and remove the fetus as soon as the diagnosis is confirmed. Often this requires removal of the tube but lately with earlier diagnosis, techniques have been developed to save the tube. More about this and ectopics in general on pages 209–10. Just be sure and report any bleeding or cramping. It may be nothing but it also may be very important.

○○○○○○○○○○○○○ **THINGS TO THINK ABOUT** ○○○○○○○○○○○○○

Your primelife pregnancy is very definitely planned and wanted. Therefore, you are probably listening to and following your doctor's advice pretty closely and altering your life-style somewhat if it was not already temple-oriented. You want a healthy full-term baby and you certainly want it to have a healthy mother. You have been reading and hearing a great deal about the effects that your mature years can have on reproduction. You have also noted the reports on special tests and procedures now available to help protect you both. Still, your mature years and your readings give you cause for concern and you ask yourself—am I going to have a damaged or slow-to-learn infant, or worse, just because I waited until now to get pregnant? Consider, then, the following:

> ○ The incidence of congenital malformations is increasing each year—worldwide. No one knows exactly why. But increasing likewise is the worldwide consumption of alcohol. Alcohol is the most common and most readily available teratogen (malformation producer).

∘ While there is an incredible and constant outcry accompanied by great thunder and immense legal efforts to protect born and unborn infants from abuse and worse (the Baby Doe principle, for instance), the tobacco industry continues to direct heavy advertising to women of childbearing age ("You've come a long way, baby"). Now, an average mother who smokes subjects her unborn child to 27,000 chemical insults (inhalations) during pregnancy, robbing it of oxygen and polluting it with poisons that permanently arrest its growth and mental development. Proven. The manufacturers must admit it now on their packaging and in their advertising.

∘ In some of our states, the *leading* cause of maternal death and of stillbirths has absolutely nothing to do with pregnancy, obstetrical care, or maternal age. The cause of this tragic loss is automobile accidents! Most of these deaths are preventable by the use of seat belts which are standard equipment on all cars and which are required by law to be buckled in many progressive states—but often aren't.

∘ Malnutrition is the leading cause of prematurity and fetal wastage in our country. Malnutrition is very often related not to poverty but to habits.

∘ In our "liberated" society, sexually transmitted diseases are about to destroy us. Many of these diseases have severe—even fatal—fetal implications.

Now, look hard at that list. These are all *nonobstetrical* factors and have *nothing* to do with calendar years of the mother. They *vastly* outweigh any other problems that might befall you because of the calendar. They are almost *totally* within your grasp to control.

∘∘∘∘∘∘∘

Hyperemesis gravidarum—vomiting of pregnancy—has been described in medical records for at least 4000 years. Only headaches have a longer medical pedigree. Here are some more things about hyperemesis:

∘ Pregnant women afflicted with this disorder generally do not abort. Their babies are not small for dates, and do not suffer intrauterine growth retardation (see pages 133–34) even if intravenous feeding has been necessary in early pregnancy.

   ○ Vomiting most often occurs in first-time mothers who are under twenty and often uneducated. Apparently women who weigh over 170 pounds are also at greater risk. Some experts say that if you vomit in one pregnancy, you will likely do so in the next. I disagree with that statement, and I go a ways back. No 4000 years, but far enough!

○ ○ ○ ○ ○ ○ ○

Toxins in the work place. The extent to which occupational exposure in American workers produces adverse reproductive outcomes is largely unknown, according to the communicable disease center's birth defect monitoring program. Further, it is believed that the problem is both widespread and serious. Research in this area is in its infancy and there must be a continuing effort to elucidate the work place causes of adverse reproductive outcomes. Thus, the list of known reproductive dangerous manufacturing chemicals as listed in this book may be far from complete but it is the best that I can obtain.

○ ○ ○ ○ ○ ○ ○

The incidence of ectopic (tubal) pregnancy has doubled in the last ten years. This tragic epidemic has been largely due to two factors now influencing primelife mothers. First, there has been a phenomenal explosion in the incidence of sexually transmitted diseases. Such diseases tend to damage normal tubal function in women and thus the pregnancy is more likely to come to rest in a tube rather than in the uterus. Second, for reasons as yet unknown, ectopic pregnancy has increased fourfold among women who smoke. Although the mortality from ectopic pregnancy has declined in a dramatic slide recently, the *greatest* incidence of occurrence has been—and still is—among women *over* thirty-five.

○ ○ ○ ○ ○ ○ ○

A human fetus, as you know, is generally accepted to be an allograft upon its mother. An allograft is human tissue of the same species but with a different genetic makeup, which is grafted onto another person. The host mother's immune tissue recognizes the fetus as such, and, as would be expected, her immune system mounts an attack upon this foreign graft. Mothers who do not possess adequate blocking antibodies that are capable of neutralizing such an attack may habitually abort. Much research is being conducted in this area.

As our worldwide experience grows in the use of frozen embryos, which can be preserved and implanted years later, the implications of the allograft principle will soon be upon us morally, ethically, and legally. The legal ramifications alone are frightening to contemplate. If the courts continue to hold that a fetus is in fact a graft, then the nonviable infant will have the same rights as any other organ transplant—no more, no less. Thus, when a conflict arises, all decisions will be made by the pregnant woman.

○○○○○○○○○○○○○○○○○○○○○○○○○○○○○○○○○○○○○○○○○○

# ∘ 2 ∘

# Basic Considerations

## EXERCISE

The United States Public Health Service has designated physical fitness as important in improving public health. It further states:

∘ Only 20 percent of American adults engage in sufficient physical activity to promote cardiovascular fitness.

∘ Leisure time physical activity is more likely to involve men than women.

∘ The higher the income bracket, the greater the fitness activity.

∘ Participation is inversely associated with age.

∘ Although we are eating *less* than our counterparts of the 1900's, we weigh *more*. Decreased physical activity is the culprit.

Women are increasingly asking their obstetricians about exercising during pregnancy—and rightly so. Many of them are already involved in fitness programs and have an excellent understanding of the basic principles of the physiology of exercise. But obviously, more need to be involved. Here are some energy facts:

◦ Short bursts of muscle activity are achieved by energy stored within muscles—about ten seconds' worth.

◦ Subsequent energy is provided by burning sugar without oxygen—anaerobic glycolysis. This system lasts longer than the first, but eventually produces cramps and fatigue. It also produces as a by-product lactic acid, which can be harmful to a fetus.

◦ Aerobic muscle metabolism is the third method of producing energy and it depends upon delivering oxygen to the muscles rapidly and regularly for sustained activity as well as physiological balance, and this requires regular, meaningful exercise.

Now what about energy, exercise, and pregnancy? Here are the salient points:

◦ Meaningful exercise standards for pregnant women have not yet been set. Most of them are intuitive. As a result, exercise programs supposedly designed for pregnant and postpartum women are largely inappropriate. Studies show that 40 percent of nonpregnant women sustain significant injuries in exercise classes as do 75 percent of their instructors.

◦ No evidence exists to show that regular exercise will improve the outcome of pregnancy—neither the quality of labor nor the fetal outcome. There is accumulating evidence that *excessive* exercise produces significant fetal hazards.

◦ During pregnancy, the following important physiological changes take place:

Connective tissue becomes softer and thus joints and tissue become more susceptible to injury.

The blood volume increases dramatically and during exercise the blood supply to the brain and the heart remains constant, but it is diverted away from major abdominal organs and this includes the uterus and therefore the fetus. This can be particularly dangerous if anemia (low red blood cell count) is also present.

Respiratory ventilation decreases and pulmonary reserve cannot always compensate for exercise and so the risk of lactic acid accumulation increases.

Nutritional needs during pregnancy includes 300 extra calories a day and much more for very active women. These needs must be met to avoid weight loss, and again, acidosis.

Dehydration (water loss) and heat loss are both much more likely to take place during pregnancy due to a number of changes, not the least of which is the increased body surface. These two conditions can very quickly and very seriously alter fetal well-being.

Blood sugar levels can fall very rapidly during pregnancy and at a much greater rate while exercising strenuously.

Fetal activity is reflected by maternal exercise activity. This includes changes in fetal heart and respiratory rate as well as fetal movements.

Based on the information above and other considerations, the following recommendations have been formulated by the American College of Obstetricians and Gynecologists:*

## Pregnancy only

º Maternal heart rate should not exceed 140 beats per minute.

º Strenuous activities should not exceed fifteen minutes in duration.

º No exercise should be performed on one's back after the fourth month of gestation is completed.

º Exercises that employ the Valsalva maneuver should be avoided (increasing intrachest pressure by forced exhalation).

º Caloric intake should be adequate to meet not only the extra energy needs of pregnancy, but also of the exercise performed.

º Maternal core temperature should not exceed 38° (100.4 F.).

*American College of Obstetricians and Gynecologists, *Exercise During Pregnancy and the Postnatal Period* (ACOG Home Exercise Programs). Washington, D.C.: ACOG, 1985.

## Pregnancy and postpartum

o Regular exercise (at least three times per week) is preferable to intermittent activity. Competitive activities should be discouraged.

o Vigorous exercise should not be performed in hot, humid weather or during a period of febrile illness.

o Ballistic movements (jerky, bouncy motions) should be avoided. Exercise should be done on a wooden floor or a tightly carpeted surface to reduce shock and provide a sure footing.

o Deep flexion or extension of joints should be avoided because of connective tissue softening. Activities that require jumping, jarring motions or rapid changes in direction should be avoided because of joint instability.

o Vigorous exercise should be preceded by a five-minute period of muscle warm-up. This can be established by slow walking or stationary cycling with low resistance.

o Vigorous exercise should be followed by a period of gradually declining activity that includes gentle stationary stretching because connective tissue softening increases the risk of joint injury. Stretches should not be taken to the point of maximum resistance.

o Heart rate should be measured at times of peak activity. Target heart rates and limits established in consultation with a physician should not be exceeded.

o Care should be taken to rise gradually from the floor to avoid orthostatic hypotension. Some form of activity involving the legs should be continued for a brief period.

o Liquids should be taken liberally before and after exercise to prevent dehydration. It necessary, activity should be interrupted to replenish fluids.

o Women who have led sedentary life-styles should begin with physical activity of a very low intensity and advance activity levels very gradually.

o Activity should be stopped and the physician consulted if any unusual symptoms appear.

# RISK FACTORS AND EXERCISE

## Relative contraindications

Your physician will need to evaluate you individually with respect to an exercise program. The following conditions may mean that vigorous physical activity during pregnancy should be avoided:

- Hypertension
- Anemia or other blood disorders
- Thyroid disease
- Diabetes
- Cardiac arrhythmia or palpitations
- History of precipitous labor
- History of intrauterine growth retardation (IUGR)
- History of bleeding during present pregnancy
- Breech presentation in the last trimester
- Excessive obesity
- Extreme underweight
- History of extremely sedentary life-style

## Absolute contraindications

The following conditions are considered absolute contraindications to vigorous exercise during pregnancy:

- History of three or more spontaneous abortions
- Ruptured membranes
- History of premature labor
- Diagnosed multiple gestation
- Incompetent cervix
- Bleeding or a diagnosis of placenta previa
- Diagnosed cardiac disease

You must be aware, of course, that complications arising during pregnancy may contraindicate vigorous activity even if you were previously able to exercise without restriction.

## Bottom line for primelifers

Continuation of an exercise program within the above guidelines offers maintenance of muscle tone and cardiovascular reserve, continuation of a positive self-image and mood levels, and reduced risk of back disorders.

In a normal pregnancy, exercise programs that follow the basic guidelines should only be discontinued if the already listed warning signs appear. Reasonable exercise in late pregnancy appears to be safe. Get your personal obstetrician's blessing early on. You may have a little clinker in your program or in your personal health of which you are unaware.

The American College of Obstetricians and Gynecologists offers the best videotape exercise program for pregnancy. Write:

American College of Obstetricians and Gynecologists (Educational Department)
Suite 300, 600 Maryland Avenue, S.W.
Washington, D.C. 20024


## SPORTS

Of course, there is great positive value in sporting activity: competition, challenge, exertion, conquest—even defeat—all of these things and more that flow from pure uncomplicated sports activity help to fill out a life and personality as can few other events. During your primelife pregnancy, some sporting guidelines must be considered. Weighed against the general benefits already listed, plus the variable exercise values, depending upon the sport involved, is some degree of general pregnancy risk.

In certain activities your risk of injury is substantially greater because as you know, your joints are now more loosely put together and easier to strain, your footing and balance is not secure, and you have an increased tendency to heat up the body and to lose fluids more rapidly over a larger skin area.

For these reasons and certain others in special situations to be covered, some restrictions are advisable for everyone's well-being. Here are considerations for specific sports:

o Hunting and fishing. Here, for example, are two fairly benign and very common sports, but supposing you're going fishing and the wind is up and your companion is a moron turned loose with a 100 horsepower motor on a twelve-foot canoe. Or say you are hunting and your shotgun has a recoil factor of a sidewinder missile? See what I mean? Take care in special situations and make sure that you are following your general exercise guidelines rather than Rambo's.

o Tennis, golf, bowling. No problems in the main. But remember, your fingers may swell in late pregnancy and they can get stuck in your bowling ball.

o Water sports. Swimming is excellent as is snorkeling. Scuba diving should be avoided because of potential placental problems that have been detected under the intense pressure of relatively shallow dives.

o Water skiing. This poses only the risk of injury—something that can happen in any sport.

o Snow sports. Skiing poses certain real hazards other than just injury. Most often you arrive at the high altitudes of ski resorts by plane and thus are suddenly dumped into a low oxygen tension atmosphere. This is hard on you and even more so on your baby. You should avoid any real physical activity for twenty-four—and preferably forty-eight—hours while your system adjusts. Otherwise, your baby may have a real oxygen deficit. If, of course, you already live as high above sea level as your ski resort, then you need not restrict yourself. There aren't many places in the United States that are that high. For instance, Denver is about 5000 feet above sea level, but Aspen Village, 120 miles away, is 3000 feet higher.

o Snowmobiles. They should be avoided.

o Softball. A popular sport for both sexes in this part of the world. It is somewhat dangerous for potential injury as well as for fluid loss and overheating. Better to be team manager.

o Competitive sports. Sports involving regular training and stressful exercises, e.g., Olympic competition, are out. There is real danger to the pregnancy.

These are largely, then, just some of the popular sports. Tae kwon do, bullfighting, and scaling Everest are your own decisions to make! Basically, however, it is well established that the benefits of regular sporting activity are such that they outweigh many of the risks—pregnant or not. Remember, though, that risks do exist, and that you and/or your baby may be hurt in almost any of them. Sport with care.

And remember, sports involving sudden changes in height and/or sudden tension on the body (flying unpressurized, tree flying, skydiving, scuba, tower diving) all can have serious fetal effects.

## HOBBIES

About 70,000,000 of us are caught up by some spare-time activity that is creative, self-fulfilling, and rewarding. Of course, most usual hobbies are safe at all times, but pregnancy does impose certain limits on some of them. The hobbies which must be reassessed during pregnancy are those associated in their performance with certain chemicals of dubious safety. Thus:

○ Painting. Covering walls, windows, and woodwork with colorful pigment is not always a hobby and may be forced upon you. Avoid lead-based paints, spray paints (because of the propellants), and keep latex-based paints away from your skin and mouth. They generally contain mercury as a preservative.

○ If picture painting is your hobby, pigments derived from heavy metals such as lead, cadmium, and barium are toxic. Skin contact should be avoided and don't hold brushes in your mouth.

○ Sculpture, pottery. Noxious fumes are present in working in these areas, particularly in glazing. Work in a well-ventilated place or not at all.

○ Woodworking. Again, ventilation is the key. Sawdust and asbestos both can accumulate in woodworking areas.

○ Miniatures. The construction of model airplanes, cars, etc., requires certain volatile glues. These contain chemicals that are not safe during pregnancy.

○ Photography. Take pictures, but stay out of the dark-room. Chemicals again.

○ Gardening. The problem here again is chemicals. Read the label of any agent you use and then consult the section of this book dealing with chemicals in the work place.

○ Jewelry making. Cadmium is present in silver solder and is highly toxic.

○ Silk screen printing. Solvent-based inks used here are involved in many toxic reactions and have been incriminated in spontaneous abortions.

Some hobbies such as scuba diving and flying are also sports and that is where they are mentioned.

## PETS

The rewards found in an animal-human bond are very sub-stantial indeed. The therapeutic and emotional support value of such bonds are very real and are well documented. But the rela-tionship, however valued, must be reexamined during pregnancy because many of our animal or avian friends are host to disorders that can be injurious at this time.

## Dogs

Dogs are the most common household pets and there are 1,100,000 registered dogs (cocker spaniels lead the list), with 4.5 million more unregistered mixtures wandering about. If you own a dog—whether it's registered or just one of the gang—you will want to keep its vaccinations and examinations current—for its sake and for yours. Dogs are a go-between that bring a number of pests into your life.

○ Ticks and fleas. There are many kinds of ticks that infest dogs in the summer, crawling into their underbodies from the ground. Most ticks are harmless even though they may attach to you and steal some blood.

Two ticks can cause harm in pregnancy. One carries tula-remia (Rocky Mountain spotted fever) which can make you very ill and can endanger your pregnancy. The other carries

a spirochete that can produce Lyme disease, a systemic illness with skin, heart, and neurological manifestations. Recently, nineteen cases were identified and five of these had
severe adverse fetal outcomes. Your land can be treated to
prevent tick infestations.

Fleas in this country are no longer vectors of dangerous
illnesses. They are merely an irritant that your dog gets from
the ground or from other animals, and carries to your carpet-
ing where they set up housekeeping for life. They pass the
time by biting your legs when there is nothing else to do. Ways
of exterminating fleas are a major source of conversation
among householders who keep pets.

○ Worms. All kind of worms can infest your dog. Proper
veterinary care can detect and get rid of most of them
promptly. Dogs frequently get pinworms, which are harmless
but which soon affect the animal's whole adopted family. Thus,
the usual treatment is administered to all family members at
the same time—this treatment, of course, includes the dog. If a
primelife mother should be involved in this scenario, she must
decline the treatment given to the rest of her family because
the medication is not known to be safe in pregnancy. The only
symptom of pinworms is irritation around the rectum (particularly during the nighttime when irritation is least needed). An
untreated mother may continue to reinfect the rest of the
family until her worms can be treated after delivery. Best
advice: regular doggy visits to the vet for a worm check.

○ Rabies. Your own dog is surely vaccinated against rabies and gets regular booster shots according to the recommendations of your veterinarian. Other dogs may not be so
protected and should you sustain a bite from a stray uniden-
tified dog, you must follow the guidelines given a few para-
graphs on ahead.

## Cats

Regardless of what social category your own cat is a member
of, it has varying chances of harboring the following:

○ Cat fever. Most cats carry, as a regular resident in their
mouths and on their claws, a bacteria that, if inoculated into

a human by a bite or a scratch, will produce an often severe illness that is characterized by fever, lymph gland enlargement, and malaise. It may resemble tularemia, plague, or even early AIDS, but, of course, is none of these.

° Toxoplasmosis. This illness, not uncommon in cats, can have very serious consequences during pregnancy. It is described in detail on page 125.

° Rabies and plague. Cats are hunters and predators by instinct. If they come across a rodent infected with plague then they may become a vector for that very dangerous disease. Plague exists in ever wider areas of the United States. If the cat's prey happens to be bats, skunks, infected dogs or cats, raccoons, or foxes, then rabies is a distinct possibility.

How best to manage your cat:

° Be sure all necessary shots are given and current.

° Keep cats out of the kitchen, don't let them lick your face, avoid bites and scratches. Do not attend to their litter boxes.

° If you give them meat, particularly pork or lamb, be sure it has been well cooked.

° Don't pet outside cats.

## Other pets

Unless you keep person-eating piranhas, fish are generally safe "pets." Exotic birds, too, are safe, provided they have been legally imported and documented. Do not make pets of any wild animals and do not try to approach any—from a chipmunk to a bear.

## Rabies

° Rabies is not an uncommon animal disease in this country. The most common rabid animal on the East Coast and in the Southeast is the raccoon. In the central United States, skunks are the leader, and in the West, it's the bats. There has never been in the United States a known human case of rabies contracted from rodents (squirrels, rats, and mice). Horses, cows, and foxes are, along with cats and dogs, other real and potential rabies carriers in this country.

o If bitten by a dog or cat of unknown vaccination status, see your doctor at once for wound treatment. If the animal is available it must be quarantined for ten days. If it is still well, no postexposure treatment for rabies is needed. Animals other than cats and dogs must be sacrificed at once and their heads sent to the state health department. Any vet can do this. If tests are negative, no rabies treatment is indicated.

o Postexposure treatment is now much simpler and safer. The vaccines and immune globulins are always available at state health offices. Any pregnant mother with a confirmed rabid bite must be treated. The benefits far outweight the risks to a pregnancy.

## WEIGHT AND NUTRITION

Note:

One chocolate eclair equals 500 calories.
Fifty pounds weight gain in pregnancy equals personal disaster!

Here are some facts about weight and pregnancy:

o Although height-adjusted average weight tables are available everywhere except on public bathroom walls, the table on page 46 is reproduced here for you to use as a guide. If 85 percent below normal, you are underweight, and above 120 percent you are overweight—and more weight than that makes you obese, which is an ugly but effective word.

o At full term it is desirable, if possible, that you weigh 120 percent of your normal weight and that about four days after delivery you weigh 110 percent of normal. Women in this framework most likely will deliver infants with a normal weight and without evidence of malnutrition.

## HEIGHT AND WEIGHT TABLES

Weights at ages 25–29 based on lowest mortality. Weight in pounds according to frame (in indoor clothing weighing 5 lbs. for men and 3 lbs. for women; shoes with 1″ heels).

| MEN | | | | | WOMEN | | | | |
|---|---|---|---|---|---|---|---|---|---|
| Height Feet | Inches | Small Frame | Medium Frame | Large Frame | Height Feet | Inches | Small Frame | Medium Frame | Large Frame |
| 5 | 2 | 128–134 | 131–141 | 138–150 | 4 | 10 | 102–111 | 109–121 | 118–13 |
| 5 | 3 | 130–136 | 133–143 | 140–153 | 4 | 11 | 103–113 | 111–123 | 120–13 |
| 5 | 4 | 132–138 | 135–145 | 142–156 | 5 | 0 | 104–115 | 113–126 | 122–13 |
| 5 | 5 | 134–140 | 137–148 | 144–160 | 5 | 1 | 106–118 | 115–129 | 125–14 |
| 5 | 6 | 136–142 | 139–151 | 146–164 | 5 | 2 | 108–121 | 118–132 | 128–14 |
| 5 | 7 | 138–145 | 142–154 | 149–168 | 5 | 3 | 111–124 | 121–135 | 131–14 |
| 5 | 8 | 140–148 | 145–157 | 152–172 | 5 | 4 | 114–127 | 124–138 | 134–15 |
| 5 | 9 | 142–151 | 148–160 | 155–176 | 5 | 5 | 117–130 | 127–141 | 137–15 |
| 5 | 10 | 144–154 | 151–163 | 158–180 | 5 | 6 | 120–133 | 130–144 | 140–15 |
| 5 | 11 | 146–157 | 154–166 | 161–184 | 5 | 7 | 123–136 | 133–147 | 143–16 |
| 6 | 0 | 149–160 | 157–170 | 164–188 | 5 | 8 | 126–139 | 136–150 | 146–16 |
| 6 | 1 | 152–164 | 160–174 | 168–192 | 5 | 9 | 129–142 | 139–153 | 149–17 |
| 6 | 2 | 155–168 | 164–178 | 172–197 | 5 | 10 | 132–145 | 142–156 | 152–17 |
| 6 | 3 | 158–172 | 167–182 | 176–202 | 5 | 11 | 135–148 | 145–159 | 155–17 |
| 6 | 4 | 162–176 | 171–187 | 181–207 | 6 | 0 | 138–151 | 148–162 | 158–17 |

Source of basic data: 1979 Build Study, Society of Actuaries and Association of Life Insurance Medical Directors of America, 1980. Copyright 1983 Metropolitan Life Insurance Company.

° The average desirable weight gain in pregnancy is 23–29 pounds, distributed as follows:

| | |
|---|---|
| Expanded maternal blood volume | 2 lbs. |
| Breast enlargement | 3–4 |
| Uterine expansion | 1–2 |
| "Lactation" fat deposits | 7–10 |
| Fetus | 8 |
| Amniotic fluid | 1 |
| Placenta | 1–2 |
| Total | 23–29 |

° Weight gain in the first three months should be slight. Then there is a steady addition of just under one pound per week thereafter.

○ The fetal compartment (fetus, amniotic fluid, and placenta) comprises about eleven pounds at full term, the remainder going to the maternal compartment. Most of the maternal compartment is filled in the first and second trimester while the third belongs mainly to the fetus.

○ To gain this much weight, the maternal diet must be increased by 300 to 400 calories per day, assuming a normal prepregnant diet of about 2000 daily calories—perhaps a dangerous assumption.

○ No pregnant woman should try to lose weight for any reason. Even obese expectants should gain at least fifteen pounds. Admittedly, as you will see later, obesity itself contributes to many serious complications of pregnancy; nonetheless, pregnancy is not the time to attack it.

○ Women who enter pregnancy underweight should do all they can to compensate for this state and increase their daily caloric intake well above 500 additional units. Sometimes as much as forty pounds must be laid down to achieve this. Significantly, underweight women have the same risk of producing a growth-retarded infant as do their overweight sisters.

○ Most developed-nation diets contain adequate calories but some specific nutritional deficiencies are not uncommon. The most usual are iron, folic acid, calcium, and zinc. Although most balanced, nutritionally sound diets can replace these substances, it is probably best to take a prenatal vitamin/mineral supplement provided by your physician. Avoid fads and excessive vitamin/mineral supplements like poison.

○ Lactation and thus breast feeding involves the loss of large amounts of nutrients. The quality of breast milk seems to be maintained across a wide variety of maternal diets and is relatively independent of maternal intakes. It does this at the expense of maternal stores unless the diet is adequate. Therefore a daily caloric intake of 2500 calories should be maintained and supplemental minerals and vitamins should be continued while breast feeding.

Some fetal facts:

- The fetus, as was once believed, cannot take from its mother and protect itself from maternal dietary deficiencies. Thus, what she lacks, it lacks.
- Even a modest maternal nutritional lack can affect the fetus—iron deficiency anemia is a good and common example.
- The *leading* cause of fetal loss is *premature* birth and its leading cause is *malnutrition*.

In general, the nutritional management of pregnancy is better understood and easier to manage today. Most women who eat enough to satisfy their appetite gain enough weight. If their diet is varied and fad-free, they get most of the vitamins and minerals they need. Nonetheless, supplements containing at least iron, folic acid, calcium, and zinc should be taken daily. No woman should try to lose weight during pregnancy and some should gain in excess of the averages established.

## DIET

Well, now, you are briefed on weight and nutrition and that roughly 2500 calories represents your needs for daily bread during pregnancy. Calories, as you probably know, are measures of the energy released by a specific food as it is oxidized in the body. And everybody knows that a raspberry torte releases more energy when it burns than, weight for weight, celery sticks. Sad but true. The caloric values of all foods are available almost everywhere that food is bought, sold, discussed, described, prepared, eaten, written about, or thought about. You may even find a list in the back of your checkbook—or in your Hallmark datebook. Most canned, frozen, or otherwise prepared foods list on their labels, among other things, the caloric values of the enclosed edibles. Finally, in your heart of hearts, you know—really know—that you can estimate the calories in just about everything you are about to scarf. You've lived long enough for that!

It is a fact of American life that we are preparing fewer and fewer of our own meals. The average American now eats out at least four times each week. It is unfortunate that some of the most popular eat-out emporiums are preparing the least nutritional meals (see Things to Think About, pages 70–71).

Moreover, many of the meals eaten at home are, of course, bought at a fast-food drive-through establishment and many of these food sources now offer delivery services. The pizza industry, for instance, is now doing more home deliveries than doctors ever dreamed of. Without much fuss, Granny Kroger will prepare your whole Christmas dinner as fast as you can tap out her number and surrender your cash.

Finally, there is a vast array of frozen meals, which of all sources of outside prepared sustenance, are most likely to list the nutritional and caloric components of the contents shivering inside. As a general rule, the lastest generation of frozen foods is nutritionally top drawer.

Because of this eat-out, buy-out, eat-in revolution, it is becoming increasingly difficult to assess caloric intake and further to be certain of the nutritional values of what we eat. Granted the present situation is probably better than when eating in meant opening a can of beef stew and a can of fruit salad for dinner, still the nutritional and caloric values of what you eat are better assessed if you eat at home more often and use fresh or frozen basic foods. If you do this, the following information will be of some value to you and your baby:

° Keep your total caloric intake at 2300 to 2500 calories daily.

° Make sure your diet consists of 50 percent carbohydrates, 25% fat, and 25% protein.

° Avoid refined sugar, which has no nutrient value at all.

° Too much of your present diet probably contains fat. Keep the fat portion of your diet to 25 percent. General guidelines: two thirds of your fat is of animal origin (meats, milk products); one third is plant (coconut, chocolate, avocado, peanut, olive, nuts, corn, soybean).

° Avoid too much red meat and get protein from fish and fowl.

Here are the four basic food groups and your daily needs from each:

○ *Milk, cheese, yogurt, ice cream.* Two eight-ounce glasses of milk or two cups of ice cream, or two ounces of cheese.

○ *Vegetables/fruit group.* One serving of fruit, one of dark green vegetable, and two of light vegetable or other fruit. Potatoes count as a light vegetable.

○ *Meat, fish, foul, eggs, legumes (soybeans, beans, peas), and nuts.* Two or more servings of three ounces (meats, etc.) or one cup cooked (legumes).

○ *Bread, cereal, rice.* Four or more servings. Bread is better as whole grained enriched. One slice equals one serving. Three quarters of a cup of rice or cooked cereal is one serving. One serving of a dried prepared cereal is defined on the package label. Read carefully.

Now, then, three meals a day works best—with each meal containing at least three of the four basic groups and with all four groups getting full attention in any one day. There are some restrictions, however.

○ Some primelife mothers may for medical reasons (hypertension, arteriosclerosis, etc.) be restricted in their intake of animal fats to a considerable degree. These dietary restrictions must be continued and the extra protein found in fish and fowl (skinned).

○ Eggs, which are neither fish, fowl, meat, nor vegetable, are generally a recommended source of protein nutrition in most diets—including pregnancy diets. Two per day is not uncommon. However, egg yolk is exceedingly high in animal fat and the daily intake of two eggs seems to be a very bad dietary habit to form at any time of life, pregnant or not. The protein is available elsewhere.

○ Milk may not be a good adult food—in fact, it probably isn't. In the first place, most adults cannot digest lactose (milk sugar). This fact leads to many adult digestive disturbances. Second, about 20 percent of all adults are allergic to milk and this leads to many other health disturbances. Third, milk fat is another fat source on the endangered or endangering list so unless it is fat-free, skimmed, and tasteless, it must be avoided by many adults. Thus other protein and calcium sources must be substituted in the diet.

° Coffee and tea are all right in limited amounts—one or two cups a day. No calories are involved. Saccharine and Nutrasweet have not been proven harmful in pregnancy.

° Alcohol, as will be seen, except in very limited amounts after the third month is a teratogen and a dangerous drug. It is also very high in "empty" calories with no food value.

° Soft drinks are harmless—unless they contain caffeine and are abused—and are a further source of empty calories. Well, look. Two cola drinks or one martini during the day provide over 300 calories—good for nothing. In order not to gain excessively, you would have to avoid a nutritious breakfast that same day—and every day in which that eating pattern is continued. Tell that to your little fellow traveler!

° Sodium is a tender subject both in medicine and nutrition. Americans generally eat tons more salt than their bodies require—some as much as 200 times their daily needs! Excess salt in the diet has been clearly linked to the onset of hypertension and all its problems. As far as obstetrics is concerned, salt at one time was thought to be the culprit in hypertension of pregnancy. That theory is no longer tolerable, but when it was, salt was almost eliminated from pregnancy diets.

If you are already hypertensive, you may be on a salt-restricted diet. If not hypertensive, you should still salt your food lightly and avoid salty foods. If you want to gain five pounds of water and blow your shoes off your feet, try a big ham dinner sometime during the last trimester.

This is just a brief outline of your diet and nutritional needs. A detailed pregnancy diet may be obtained from your local or state health departments, or, if you have years to wait, from the National Institutes of Health, Division of Human Reproduction, Rockville, MD. Or for immediate information, write to the American College of Obstetricians and Gynecologists, Suite 300, 600 Maryland Avenue S.W., Washington, D.C. 20024

## HYGIENE

Whatever your normal patterns of cleanliness involve, pregnancy is not likely to disturb most of them. But still, some must be forsaken. Special hygienic problems introduced by pregnancy include: increased perspiration, increased bodily secretions, particularly from the breasts and vagina, and greater difficulty as time advances in covering—indeed, reaching—some body areas. Right now you might see what I mean by trying to shave your legs with a pillow tied to your waist.

Restrictions that apply during pregnancy involve limited douching, avoiding excess body heat, and revamping some "articles de toilet." Let's see how these things apply.

### Skin

Your skin will generally be more moist and oily. Bathing frequently helps and there is no reason not to. Stronger antiperspirants may be needed. In late pregnancy, the skin over the abdomen and breast stretches more rapidly and you will want to use a lanolin-based skin cream several times daily to keep the resultant stretch marks (striae) to a minimum.

Fingernail and toenail clipping and painting and body shaving—all can go on as long as the parts can be seen. To say that fastidiousness and cleanliness is extra important during pregnancy is to invite a belt on the head. You know that, and you don't need a man to tell you about it.

### Hair

Cleaning your hair is no real problem—unless it always has been. You may use standard shampoos and rinses as long as you always rinse your hair *completely* after the applications. *Avoid* tints or any chemicals that have *prolonged* hair contact or that *stay* in your hair. Do not use any *dyes* and avoid inhaling the *propellants* in your hair sprays. Better to use one with a pump-type dispenser.

Your hair may change during pregnancy. It may grow faster and become less curly. The exact reverse may also occur. Shortly after delivery you may shed a carpet of scalp hair, but be of good cheer. It grows back very quickly.

## Vaginal douching

Whether or not douching is necessary, advisable, perverted, dangerous, or a device of the decadent—during pregnancy or anytime—has raised more trivial and heated comment than the order of seating at the Last Supper. Although increased vaginal secretions may make douching more desirable during pregnancy, some restrictions are necessary because the cervix softens and opens somewhat and may be easy to *enter accidentally.* It is possible to force the douche nozzle up into the cervix so that the douche liquid enters the uterus, producing a disaster. So the nozzle must be inserted into the vagina soberly, gently, and with reasonable care. Gravity flow equipment is safer than syringe douches but either type is safe *if used properly.* Water or vinegar-and-water douches are preferred over medicated ones. Douche infrequently and only as absolutely necessary, and always clear this hygienic practice with your own obstetrician.

Never douche:

> If it is painful.
> If there is any vaginal bleeding present.
> If your membranes are ruptured.
> During the last six weeks of pregnancy.
> If your doctor forbids it.

## Bathing

There are certain restrictions about bathing that need to be observed.

° Prolonged—even short—bathing in very hot water should be avoided since fetal damage can be induced by high body temperatures.

° The family hot tub can be a bacterial cauldron rather than a safe social gathering spot. Share your hot tub like your toothbrush—gingerly. And closely observe instructions for its maintenance.

° Public tubs, pools, and spas have unfortunately been shown to harbor yeast and other more serious transmissible infections, as do their surrounding stools and benches.

Except for the above circumstances, you may tub as often as you wish as long as you wish—until you cannot keep your head above water or when you can't see your feet over your tummy.

## Showering

There are no restrictions that would keep you from showering unless your shower is a tub. In that case, unless you have some firm grasping handles, showering in late pregnancy poses monumental balancing hazards that might be best avoided.

## DENTAL CARE

There has been a lot of misinformation about the fate and the care of teeth during pregnancy. To replace it, here is some first-class dental information—which, in today's rapidly changing world, may become first-class misinformation before you have another baby. In the meantime, it's the best there is.

° The calcium in your diet and in your vitamin/mineral supplement is important for bone and tooth formation in your developing infant and also to protect your own calcium needs. The calcium in your teeth, however, is not during pregnancy or any other time vulnerable to removal or loss—except by decay.

° Tooth decay is more common in pregnancy because frequent small meals—often advised in both early and late pregnancy—expose the teeth to food more frequently, thereby increasing the chances for decay, and vomiting—not unusual in early pregnancy—exposes the teeth to more acid erosion from the stomach contents.

° The gums are more likely to swell and bleed during pregnancy. This is due to hormonal changes, not to periodontal disease or vitamin C deficiency. These soft, sensitive gums are, however, more prone to develop periodontal disease if not cared for properly.

In the light of all the above, it is clear that dental hygiene and dental visits are an important part of your care, so:

° Clean and brush your teeth after each and every meal. Dental floss and water-jet devices are extremely important and should be used regularly, but with greater gentleness. You may also have to resort to a softer toothbrush.

° Avoid empty carbohydrates (see Diet, pages 48–51) in your snacks or in-between meals—they greatly increase the risk of decay.

° See your dentist early on. For a number of reasons, restorative dental work may be delayed until you are in the second trimester, but plan to seek care early anyway. And be sure to announce that you are pregnant!

° Your dentist will know that there are certain things to avoid at this time. For instance:

Some medications can affect your developing infant. These include inhalation gases, certain antibiotics (particularly tetracyclines), and some substances used with local anesthetics—although local anesthetics are themselves safe to use.

X-rays—unless very important, and unless you are shielded with a lead apron—should be avoided.

Elective dental work might better be postponed.

No matter what delays may beset you, get to your dentist while you can still lie back in his chair and while your dentist can still work above your loaded abdomen.

## SEX

There exists a limited school of scientists who believe sex should be avoided entirely during pregnancy. According to this belief, sex at this time is dangerous for two reasons:

° The physical and emotional stimulation of sexual activity may induce an abortion or premature labor.

° The uterine cervix is increasingly sensitive to certain irritants during pregnancy—one of them being certain viruses often present on men's genitals. Such irritation, they postulate, may increase the likelihood of cervical cancer in later years.

There is some truth to both contentions and more will be said about the first when we discuss premature labor. As far as the second is concerned, much remains to be learned in this speculative area.

Sufficient to say for now is that, as far as we know, sexual activity of considerable variety appears safe and desirable in a normal pregnancy, and there is not much that will stop it. There are, however, some altered ground rules.

## Vaginal penetration

This is the end point as well as the in-between point in most sexual encounters. Vaginal penetration should be avoided:

- If it produces pain—at any stage of pregnancy.
- When there is any vaginal bleeding of any kind with or without pain.
- If a vaginal infection exists.
- If the membranes are ruptured.
- During the last weeks of pregnancy—or much earlier if there is a history of premature labor.
- If your physician says so—or says no, rather.

## Foreplay

This area of lovemaking is very personal and involves many variable likes and dislikes. Do what you have been enjoying but note that:

- Breast suckling may be tender at times and may produce a secretion that is very slightly bitter to the taste—his. Breast suckling is dangerous in late pregnancy—particularly if there is a substantial history of premature labor. See page 269.
- Oral-genital loving creates no problems unless infection is present. Personal fastidiousness is very important since secretions are heavier even without infection.
- Blowing into the vagina is not an uncommon form of foreplay. It must, however, be avoided during pregnancy.

° Anal penetration must be avoided during pregnancy. The rectum is a tender spot as the pressure above increases and too much bacterial contamination can result from anal sojourns.

° No ice, hot water, or internal vibrators.

## Some general points

° Closeness, understanding, and warmth is important. This is a tender, brittle, emotional time for both. Be considerate of each other's needs.

° Sexual desires may be altered—one way or the other the alterations need to be respected.

° During orgasm women may experience sharp menstrual-like cramps. These are not dangerous, and will not normally start labor.

° Any position that is rewarding and comfortable is a good position. As the baby grows, alternate approaches to vaginal penetration are more comfortable.

° Again, vaginal penetration should absolutely be no more when:

It's not pleasant.
The membranes are ruptured.
The doctor says no.

° Mutual masturbation by whatever means is a reasonable and safe alternative to vaginal penetration anytime.

In a recent study on sexuality during and after pregnancy, it was found, for the most part, that women's sexual appetite declines markedly as pregnancy advances, but usually returns to previous levels after birth. The frequency and quality of orgasm declines slightly as pregnancy advances and remains low for about three months after delivery. Regardless of instructions, about one quarter continued sexual activity during the last weeks of pregnancy—even into early labor. About half abstained from three to six weeks before labor and the remainder as early as three months. The reasons for cessation were lack of interest, not advice! Many couples were able to achieve mutual orgasm without vaginal penetration both before and after delivery. Finally, unplanned pregnancies were significantly associated with diminished sexual desire during pregnancy, but not after birth.

## SHOWING

Showing takes place at different times in different pregnancies all depending upon:

○ Previous pregnancies. Once you have been stretched, it is easier—and quicker—to stretch again.

○ Body build. Showing occurs when the growing uterus itself, or the organs it has pushed up into your abdomen, or both together reach such a size that something has to give. And the easiest thing to give is the old front wall—your tummy. It gives. You show. But if you have a deep, full pelvic bowl, you may be able to contain all the new material longer than someone with a tiny pelvic bowl. So anatomy counts.

○ Twins, triplets, and on up, of course, show sooner.

○ Your beginning weight and girth. Obviously, if you have a well-endowed abdominal substance to begin with, you can conceal a pregnancy for a much longer period of time, whether you want to or not.

## CLOTHING

Data concerning women's clothing during pregnancy is hard to come by. Physicians are not very interested in writing about it and fashion magazines change styles too fast to record in a book. While writing this book, I asked several patients what they were most comfortable in. One said bed, another said a bath blanket, and still another, limbo. So that source wasn't much help either.

The best era for pregnant women so far as styles are concerned was the time of the shift, a hollow cloth tube with openings at both ends and no gather in the middle. You could slip it over the top or pull it up from the bottom. Women were dressed not only in style but were quite comfortable throughout pregnancy. The fact that many nonpregnant women looked pregnant probably contributed to an early death of the shift. Recent styles appear to favor loose-fitting shirts and sweaters and would seem to offer much comfortable room for pregnant women to stretch in as things progress. Hopefully—but not likely—they will be around for a while.

But now to the nitty-gritty—let's take it from the top.

○ Do you have to wear a bra while pregnant? No, you don't. Nor do you have to wear shoes to work, but you will be much more comfortable both shod and uplifted. Breasts become congested and swollen at this time and generally grow heavier as pregnancy continues. A significant strain is placed upon the tissue bands which support your breasts and, without help, they may be damaged, and support gone. Moreover, breast secretions begin early on and, without a bra, may stain whatever stands between them and the world. Sometimes a nursing shield is necessary for further protection even with the thickest of bras. Finally, irritation of the nipples may cause painful uterine contractions at any time and at full term may even start labor! Don't laugh. This fact has several other important ramifications, some of which may come readily to mind. See breast stimulation test, page 269. So, it might be better to knuckle down and fasten up. It is still, however, a very personal decision.

○ Waistline. It makes good sense to keep your waistline fairly loose and comfortable. It seems to me that I read recently that bodices and corsets were on the way back. I hope that is not so—and you can forget about them! Sometimes a girdle of sorts is necessary to protect certain back problems— this is rarely the case, however. Pelvic tilt exercises are much better in most back problems. Your doctor will know.

Your waistline will probably be the key that turns you into maternity clothes. Your growing pregnancy starts protruding into your abdomen during the second trimester but it may have already pushed other organs on up above and out of its way, thus providing you with a mound where there was once a plateau. Many variables can alter the time when all this begins to appear on your tape measure (muscle strength, previous pregnancies, multiple pregnancies [twins +], and so forth). But get into your new garments early rather than struggling to put down a front. Safety pins are only so safe and can only hold your pants together so long! Although you may be ready to shred and burn your maternity clothes at the end, at least they have carried you there in comfort.

   o Panties. Most bottoms are protected today by nylon garments—which is fine except that during pregnancy there is a good deal more moisture, secretions, and heat generated in the vaginal area. Nylon tends to trap all this activity and, if further overcoated by nylon pantyhose, clearly produces a formidable barrier. Thus there is an increased likelihood of local skin irritation and perhaps infections such as yeast. Cotton panties and pantyhose with cotton crotches may be the answer. In case you should develop signs of vaginitis— itching, redness, and swelling—you must consult your doctor.

   Abundant and attractive maternity swimsuits are available and you should swim as often as you can—all things being equal. After you finish swimming, get out of your suit to prevent irritation, shower thoroughly, and sun in something dry. And although this is beginning to sound like an endless lecture, your tolerance to sunlight is decreased, so watch it.

   o Pantyhose have been mentioned above. Pregnancy pantyhose and support pantyhose are available everywhere and should be used when needed. Never wear hose with leg garters or other leg-constricting support. Your leg circulation is taxed enough as it is.

   o Shoes. Okay, I agree. The only shoes for pregnant women that would satisfy all doctors are British walking Braughams—which, if they weighed a little less, could be used to walk on water. But there are reasonable compromises. Your feet take a beating during pregnancy because of increased body weight, changes in posture, loosening of ligaments, swelling, and increase in foot size.

   Therefore, be good to them. Don't wear high heels, or unstable shoes, or tight shoes, or heavy shoes, or toeless shoes, or nonsupportive shoes. Somewhere in there is a compromise that looks good and feels good. Your foot size may go up by one size during pregnancy—maybe.

Narrow, pointed, and very high-heeled shoes increase the risk of bunions, corns, calluses, ingrown toenails, hammertoes, and backaches.

If you have read all of the above, you may decide that the lady who wanted to stay in a bath blanket was right.

## BABY JITTERS

As any of you who have already had ultrasound procedures can testify, babies begin to move about very early in their careers—somewhere between the second and third month. The fetal heart is moving and pulsating and can be seen doing so as early as the seventh week. Truly amazing to behold.

Pulsations and activity of the fetal heart can probably never be felt, but fetal movements certainly can be felt and are anxiously awaited by all primelife mothers. Such movements are first noticeable at a variety of times in different pregnancies, all dependent upon:

○ Previous maternal experience. Once you've felt movement, you are more attuned to it in subsequent pregnancies.

○ Fetal personality. Some are slow movers and some are earth shakers—just like people.

○ Maternal fat insulation. Enough said on that.

○ Multiple or single infants.

No matter what, you will feel some light fluttering, like a gas bubble before the end of the fourth month, and even then, if you don't, your obstetrician will let you listen to the heartbeat on a monitor. Such happy sounds should serve to reassure you. Nothing, however, is as reassuring as that thing that goes bump in the night—night after night after night.

Later on in your pregnancy, your doctor may ask you to evaluate your baby's movements on a daily basis. This is often an important source of information as we shall see. For the present, the degree of activity generated by your baby in the early months is not much indication of anything except life within you—which, I think, is glorious news.

# HABITS—COBWEBS AT FIRST, CABLES AT THE END

"Habit," wrote William James over 100 years ago, "is the enormous flywheel of society. . . . It keeps the fisherman and deck hand at sea through the winter; it holds the miner in the darkness, and nails the countryman to his log cabin and his lonely farm through all the months of snow."

He has more to say: "The great thing, then . . . is to make the nervous system our ally instead of our enemy. For this we must make automatic and habitual, as early as possible, as many useful actions as we can. Guard against growing into ways that are likely to be disadvantageous to us—as we should guard against the plague."

Good advice—but we were supposed to act on this advice in our teens, not in our thirties. So, assuming you may have formed some bad habits by this time, here is some information that may help.

## Tobacco

In my lifetime I have seen smallpox, a onetime great killer and crippler, pneumonia, tuberculosis, syphilis, and many other severe and tragic public health problems come under control and in some instances (smallpox) disappear. You have seen in your lifetime rubella (German measles), rheumatic heart disease, and some types of cancer eliminated as public health problems. But during this same period of time, the two greatest health problems that we face as a nation have only increased in their insidious and malignant devastation of our people. And relief is more than a swallow or a puff away.

All drugs that produce dependence have these basic characteristics:

° They are all psychoactive—that is, they all effect the chemistry of the brain and nervous system.

° They all create dependence and lead to compulsive use.

° Abrupt withdrawal from the drug produces physiological and psychological distress.

○ There is a strong tendency to relapse—even after a period of prolonged withdrawal.

Nicotine—only *one* of the dangerous drugs in tobacco—fulfills all these criteria and the use of tobacco constitutes the most widespread example of drug dependency in this and many other countries.

More women smoke than men and thus more women die of lung cancer than men. Further, more women die of lung cancer than of breast cancer—or any other cancer for that matter. Here are some other special problems in women related to smoking:

○ The combination of oral contraceptives and tobacco leads to a much greater incidence of heart attacks in women.

○ Women who smoke are considerably less fertile.

○ Smoking induces an earlier menopause.

In pregnancy the unwilling fetus is subjected not only to nicotine, but also to carbon monoxide and other lethal gases that have an enormous impact on its well-being. Other points on child-bearing and smoking are:

○ Genetically healthy babies are more likely to abort spontaneously.

○ There is a fourfold increase in ectopic pregnancy.

○ Premature labor is a greater risk.

○ Growth-retarded babies are the rule rather than the exception.

○ There is apparently an increased risk of SIDS (Sudden Infant Death Syndrome).

○ Youngsters are slow to learn—and those who are born into a smoke-filled home end up having the majority of childhood respiratory ailments.

○ Recent evidence indicates that involuntary or side-stream exposure to a smoking environment has virtually the same damaging pregnancy effects. Thus, nonsmoking pregnant women who live or work in a tobacco-polluted environment are at equal risk as those who smoke. More employers are becoming aware of this evidence. Hopefully, so will more mates.

The bottom line: Don't smoke—stay away from those who do!

## Alcohol

It is hard to say which is the more destructive and pervasive public health problem, smoking or drinking. In the long run, it really doesn't matter which is first—they are both devastating. Some evidence of the drinking problem is provided by the fact that alcohol-impaired automobile drivers have caused 15 million injuries and 600,000 deaths in the past 25 years—and that is but a tiny segment of our alcohol-related health problems. Pregnancy represents another small segment but a very important one.

Since antiquity, there has been speculation about the possibility of alcohol causing pregnancy-related disorders. Only recently has the problem received wide scientific attention. It was in 1973 that the fetal alcohol syndrome was first described, and since that time sufficient work has been published so we can say without doubt that alcohol is recognized as a major fetal health hazard and as a leading established cause of mental retardation. It is the only fetal teratogen sold over the counter.

But does this evidence mean that you cannot take a single solitary drink while you are pregnant? It is true that throughout history women have consumed wine at dinner without harm, but new evidence suggests that reasonable guidelines should be followed for pregnancy safety.

Here are some guidelines for you—but you may need to check with your own doctor.

° Alcohol, as previously indicated, is a proven teratogen and therefore should be avoided in the first trimester.

° The fetal alcohol syndrome consists of growth retardation, central nervous system dysfunction, specific facial changes, and major organ malformations. The incidence of occurrence in the United States, Sweden, and France is about the same: 1 in 1000. Major racial and ethnic groups that consume alcohol regularly have not yet been studied in depth.

° The fetal alcohol syndrome is found in over one third of all heavy and regularly drinking mothers. In less active drinkers, the rate increases proportionate to daily alcohol consumption.

° Some recent evidence suggests that even an occasional drink has harmful fetal effects. But this evidence is as yet unsubstantial.

° It is clear, then, that there are no proven safety levels for alcohol consumption *after* the first trimester, but mothers who are not binge drinkers can probably have a drink before dinner or a glass of wine with dinner and not run any risk for their babies. After all, the rate of fetal alcohol syndrome occurrence noted above is 1 in 1000. I venture to say that 999 out of 1000 mothers are not *total* abstainers from alcohol.

Bottom line: It must be clear to even the most casual reader that I enjoy wine but detest tobacco. Nevertheless, in the adversarial society that surrounds us all and with firm safety lines as yet undrawn, I cannot recommend that you allow yourself anything beyond a sip of champagne—every other Saturday—after the first trimester.

## DRUGS: MEDICAL AND SOCIAL

Probably no area of medicine has been explored more deeply nor received more attention in recent times than the effect of drugs on pregnancy—in particular, of course, on the fetus. This includes medicinal as well as social drugs. Certain principles need to be stated at the beginning:

° The fetus is most vulnerable to anatomical damage during the first three months of its existence. That is the time when its body becomes fully structured and its organ system and limbs are laid down. Thereafter, it mainly grows and although many, many things can still damage it, structural defects are unlikely.

° Teratogens are drugs that can produce structural deformities, while clastogens are those that can damage a fetus without necessarily causing any visible sign or detectable structural change. As examples, alcohol is a teratogen and tobacco is a clastogen. Both are readily available without prescription.

◦ There is no placental barrier. Substances that get into the maternal circulation will get into the fetal circulation—sometimes quickly, sometimes in a greater concentration than the mother's.

◦ Almost all pregnant women take self-prescribed medicines other than vitamins. Many take more than just one—some as many as fifteen or twenty! All without prescriptions! About half of these drugs are taken in the first trimester.

◦ Practically no drug is recommended during pregnancy by physicians. Some are considered relatively safe for certain serious situations, such as penicillin for a dangerous bacterial infection, but there aren't many and the benefit-to-risk ratio must be explored in each situation. Sadly, some drugs known to be safe during pregnancy—and beneficial—have been withdrawn from the market because the manufacturing drug companies cannot afford the litigation that has falsely been thrust upon them.

Here follows a list of most specific drugs about which enough is known to classify them. This list is not and cannot be complete, as new data accumulates daily. Your best plan is to avoid any conceivable drug while attempting to conceive or after having conceived and check with your doctor.

## PRESCRIPTION DRUGS

### Teratogens

thalidomide (a sedative not available now in the United States)

Dilantin (a cerebral relaxant)

warfarin (an anticoagulant)

folic acid antagonist (generally present in anticancer drugs)

androgens and progestins (hormones)

diethylstilbestrol (DES, a hormone)

mercury (present in some medications)
Accutane (used to treat acne)

**Suspected Teratogens**

lithium (a psychiatric drug)
benzodiazepines (tranquilizers)
certain oral contraceptives
amphetamines (stimulants, often taken for weight control)
cortisone (an anti-inflammatory)
certain antihistamines

**Clastogens**

propranolol (an antihypertensive drug)
thiazides (diuretic drugs)
chloramphenicol (an antibiotic)
tetracyclines (antibiotics)
meprobamate (a tranquilizer)
reserpine (antihypertensive)
erythromycin (an antibiotic)
streptomycin (an antibiotic)

## OVER-THE-COUNTER DRUGS

**Proven Human Teratogens**

ethyl alcohol

**Suspected Human Teratogens**

None

**Clastogens**

aspirin
tobacco
caffeine
certain antihistamines
vitamins A, D, and K in excess

## UNDER-THE-COUNTER DRUGS

### Clastogens

Every one of them, from acid to grass

### COMMON MEDICATIONS THAT ARE PROBABLY SAFE

penicillin and certain derivatives
acetaminophen
mild narcotics, such as codeine, taken occasionally for
pain

For further information, read:

° Beatrice Krauer, M.D., Felix Krauer, M.D., and Frank
Hytten, M.D. *Drug Prescribing in Pregnancy.* New York:
Churchill Livingston, 1984. 188 pages.

° G.G. Briggs, T.W. Bodendorfer, R.K. Freeman, and S.J.
Yaffe. *Drugs in Pregnancy and Lactation: A Reference Guide to
Fetal and Neonatal Risk.* Baltimore: Williams & Wilkins, 1983.
415 pages.

## GROWTH AND DEVELOPMENT

This may be a good time to consider how the primelife embryo unfolds and develops inside you during its nine-month resi-
dency. Such consideration also provides an opportunity to
correlate such development with some of the monitoring studies
that follow its course.

All times are dated from the last menstrual period. Day one
therefore is the first day of the last period, and day 280 is the
expected date of delivery. Thus there are forty weeks—or ten
lunar months—till term. Conception, on the other hand, occurs
two weeks after the last period, so the actual duration of pregnancy is 265 days.

### FIRST TRIMESTER (1–14 WEEKS)

### Week

1  Last menstrual period
2  Conception

3   Implantation

4   Chorionic villi forming—beta HCG positive

5   First missed period

6   Brain and major organs forming. Regular PG tests positive and chorionic villi sampling may be attempted but usually deferred to week 9.

7   Eyes formed. Ultrasound shows heart beating.

8   Fetus moving. Maximum HCG levels being reached.

13   Extremities and organ structures completed. Fetus is swallowing.

## SECOND TRIMESTER (15–28 WEEKS)

**Week**

15   Significant amniotic fluid present. Amniocentesis may now be done; heart chambers visible on ultrasound; urine is voided.

16   Downy hair covers body. Fetal movement can be felt.

20   Baldness ceases to be a problem. Scalp hair is on.

24   Vernix (a waxy skin protectant) begins to form. Sex usually can be determined by ultrasound.

25–28   Fetus is viable and can live outside uterus.

28   Hiccups start. Biophysical profile (level II ultrasound) shows multitude of important factors. (See pages 259–60.)

## THIRD TRIMESTER (29–40 WEEKS)

**Week**

29   Subcutaneous fat begins to be deposited.

30   Fetus swallows, empties bladder and bowels, grasps, gasps, and breathes.

30–40   Lungs, kidneys, and digestive system reach maturity.

Women who run during pregnancy have smaller babies, less successful labors, and more cesarian sections. Women who are underweight and do not gain adequately have at least a 30 percent chance of delivering a small baby for dates. Finally, significant events that take place during pregnancy—particularly stressful events—can effect the newborn weight. Thus, unemployment, loss of spouse, serious family illness, and so on, have a significant and cumulative effect on the institution of premature labor and small-for-dates babies.

○○○○○○○

Drugs. Perhaps this area of concern has been overworked in my book, perhaps not. You have to see it to believe it. Ten percent of all pregnant women are on drugs, 40 percent of them smoke, and no one really knows for sure how many quietly drink. But the end results are there and speak for themselves. With the possible exception of tobacco, the use of abusive drugs and alcohol keeps increasing.

○○○○○○○

Sorry to keep harping on this, but it's important. Women who smoke demonstrate a higher rate of other risk behavior. This includes alcohol abuse and lack of seat belt use. While vaguely on the subject of seat belts, it has been reported that when seat belt instruction is included in prenatal classes, parent and child seat belt use after delivery increases up to 90 percent.

○○○○○○○

The National Institution on Drug Abuse estimates that one pregnant woman in ten is using cocaine.

○○○○○○○

According to the Center for Science in the Public Interest as published in their newsletter *Nutrition Action,* the five worst fast foods of 1985 were: McDonald's Chicken McNuggets and breakfast sausage biscuit, Wendy's cheese stuffed potato, Hardee's bacon cheeseburger, and Roy Roger's crescent sandwich with ham. These selections were made based on their high content of fat and sodium. They note, however, that some recently introduced fast foods are much better nutritionally: Long John Silver's baked fish and Wendy's low calorie salad dressings, for instance. (Copyright 1986 by CSPI. *Nutrition Action Healthletter* is available for $19.95 for 10 issues from the Center for Science in the Public Interest, 1501 16th Street N.W., Washington, D.C. 20036.)

○ ○ ○ ○ ○ ○ ○

Aspartame, the low caloric artificial sweetener, is said to be safe to use during pregnancy. Tests using six times the usual daily intake of this agent produced no evidence of fetal damage.

○ ○ ○ ○ ○ ○ ○

The total amount of iron needed by mother and baby during a pregnancy weighs about as much as an ordinary penny. But it is spent well and goes far.

○ ○ ○ ○ ○ ○ ○

Empty or "lone wolf" calories that contain nothing but energy are consumed by the American people—mainly as refined sugar—at the rate of *two pounds* per *person* per *week!*

○ ○ ○ ○ ○ ○ ○

There are many food myths that have surfaced off and on from the beginning. Thus one says that salmon eaten during pregnancy will make a bed wetter out of the baby; another that beer is good for nursing; another that cravings for unusual substances (chalk, clay, Vaseline, etc.) means that they are needed. These are all hogwash, which isn't a food substance either!

○ ○ ○ ○ ○ ○ ○ ○ ○ ○ ○ ○ ○ ○ ○ ○ ○ ○ ○ ○ ○ ○ ○ ○ ○ ○ ○ ○ ○ ○ ○ ○ ○ ○ ○ ○ ○

## ∘ 3 ∘

# Personal Care

## IMMUNIZATION

In 1954, there were in our country 18,308 cases of paralytic polio. That same year Jonas Salk's vaccine was finally released for general use. Initially, each doctor in the United States received three doses of the vaccine to use as he saw fit. You can imagine the problems caused by that type of distribution! But very shortly sufficient vaccine was available for all. By 1965, there were only sixty-five polio cases in the United States.

General appropriate immunization programs have probably done more to increase the length and quality of our lives than has *any* other single public health program. Don't avoid this responsibility for you and yours. Don't listen to antivaccine propaganda. Look in old cemeteries at the tombstones of little ones (and adults) taken away by polio, smallpox, diphtheria, whooping cough, typhoid, tetanus, and on and on.

The immune systems in our bodies marshal defenses against foreign substances that are introduced into our bodies—and which might destroy us. Mainly this is accomplished by the system's ability to identify a foreign protein (antigen) in the alien substance and to build another protein (antibody) which neutralizes the invader. Truly an incredible system—and it works. Destruction of the immune system—as, for example, occurs in

AIDS—lays our bodies naked before a host of bacterial enemies that ordinarily would be dealt with in a minor skirmish. Chemicals used in organ transplant surgery also—at least temporarily—drive down the immune response so that the donated organ will not be rejected. This unfortunately makes the recipient more vulnerable to bacterial invasion. Rarely does the immune system work against us while trying to protect us. Thus we may become allergic to penicillin. In pregnancy, the Rh incompatibility problem is generated by the immune system, and while not harming the mother, may be lethal to her baby (see page 121). Today, Rh vaccine has almost wiped out the Rh problem.

And so we come to vaccination and immunization during pregnancy—what can and can't be done, and what needs doing. First, there are four types of immunizing agents:

○ Toxoids. These are the chemically altered poisons which bacteria excrete. Example: tetanus toxoid.

○ Killed bacterial or viral vaccine. Example: typhoid, influenza.

○ Live virus vaccines which are made up of viral strains altered to reduce their virulence so that immunity develops without illness. Example: polio.

○ Immune globulin. This is a protein fraction of human plasma that supplies transient antibody activity to the recipient. It is helpful by producing quick, though short-term, protection. Example: hepatitis B, rabies.

Immunization during pregnancy must follow certain guidelines, which are generally covered in the table on pages 74–79. For information about the new hepatitis B vaccine not included in the table, see page 80.

Here is more information:

○ Rh vaccination should be carried out in susceptible pregnancy situations. See Rh, pages 120–23.

○ Influenza vaccination should be given during pregnancy in epidemic situations or if there is an underlying medical disorder that the flu would complicate.

○ Pregnant women traveling to or living in areas where yellow fever, cholera, plague (plague is here—right here—in

## IMMUNIZATION DURING PREGNANCY

| IMMUNIZING AGENT | RISK FROM DISEASE TO PREGNANT FEMALE | RISK FROM DISEASE TO FETUS OR NEONATE | TYPE OF IMMUNIZING AGENT | RISK FROM IMMUNIZING AGENT TO FETUS | INDICATIONS FOR IMMUNIZATION DURING PREGNANCY | DOSE SCHEDULE | COMMENTS |
|---|---|---|---|---|---|---|---|
| | | | *LIVE VIRUS VACCINES* | | | | |
| Measles | Significant morbidity, low mortality; not altered by pregnancy | Significant increase in abortion rate; may cause malformations | Live attenuated virus vaccine | None confirmed | Contraindicated (See immune globulins) | Single dose | Vaccination of susceptible women should be part of postpartum care. |
| Mumps | Low morbidity and mortality; not altered by pregnancy | Probable increased rate of abortion in 1st trimester. Questionable association of fibroelastosis in neonates | Live attenuated virus vaccine | None confirmed | Contraindicated | Single dose | |

| Disease | Effect of pregnancy on disease | Effect on fetus | Type of immunizing agent | Risk from immunizing agent | Indications for immunization during pregnancy | Dose schedule | Comments |
|---|---|---|---|---|---|---|---|
| Poliomyelitis | No increased incidence in pregnancy, but may be more severe if it does occur | Anoxic fetal damage reported; 50% mortality in neonatal disease | Live, attenuated virus (OPV) and inactivated virus (IPV) vaccine (Inactivated polio vaccine is recommended for unimmunized adults at increased risk.) | None confirmed | Not routinely recommended for adults in US, except persons at increased risk of exposure | *Primary:* 3 doses of IPV at 4–8 week intervals and a 4th dose 6–12 months after the 3rd dose 2 doses of OPV with a 6–8 week interval and a 3rd dose at least 6 weeks later, customarily 8–12 months later *Booster:* Every 5 years until 18 years of age for IPV | Vaccine indicated for susceptible pregnant women traveling in endemic areas or in other high-risk situations |
| Rubella | Low morbidity and mortality; not altered by pregnancy | High rate of abortion and congenital rubella syndrome | Live attenuated virus vaccine | None confirmed | Contraindicated | Single dose | Teratogenicity of vaccine is theoretical, not confirmed to date. Vaccination of susceptible women should be part of postpartum care. |
| Yellow Fever | Significant morbidity and mortality; not altered by pregnancy | Unknown | Live attenuated virus vaccine | Unknown | Contraindicated except if exposure unavoidable | Single dose | Postponement of travel preferable to vaccination, if possible |

# IMMUNIZATION DURING PREGNANCY (Continued)

| IMMUNIZING AGENT | RISK FROM DISEASE TO PREGNANT FEMALE | RISK FROM DISEASE TO FETUS OR NEONATE | TYPE OF IMMUNIZING AGENT | RISK FROM IMMUNIZING AGENT TO FETUS | INDICATIONS FOR IMMUNIZATION DURING PREGNANCY | DOSE SCHEDULE | COMMENTS |
|---|---|---|---|---|---|---|---|
| | | | *TOXOIDS* | | | | |
| Tetanus-Diphtheria | Severe morbidity; tetanus mortality 60%, diphtheria mortality 10%; unaltered by pregnancy | Neonatal tetanus mortality 60% | Combined tetanus-diphtheria toxoids preferred: adult tetanus-diphtheria formulation | None confirmed | Lack of primary series, or no booster within past 10 years | *Primary:* 2 doses at 1- to 2-month interval with a 3rd dose 6–12 months after the second; *Booster:* single dose every 10 years, after completion of the primary series | Updating of immune status should be part of antepartum care. |
| | | | *IMMUNE GLOBULINS: HYPERIMMUNE* | | | | |
| Hepatitis B | Possible increased severity during 3rd trimester | Possible increase in abortion rate and prematurity. Neonatal hepatitis can occur if mother is a chronic carrier or is acutely infected | Hepatitis B immune globulin (HBIG) | None reported | Postexposure prophylaxis | .06ml/kg immediately and 1 month later of HBIG | Infants born to HBsAg-positive mothers should receive 0.5 ml of HBIG as soon after birth as possible and the same dose repeated 3 and 6 months later. |

| Disease | Risk to mother | Risk to fetus/neonate | Immune globulin/vaccine | Adverse effects of vaccine | Indications | Dose | Comments |
|---|---|---|---|---|---|---|---|
| Rabies | Near 100% fatality; not altered by pregnancy | Determined by maternal disease | Rabies immune globulin (RIG) | None reported | Postexposure prophylaxis | 20 IU/kg in one dose of RIG | Used in conjunction with rabies killed virus vaccine |
| Tetanus | Severe morbidity; mortality 60% | Neonatal tetanus mortality 60% | Tetanus immune globulin (TIG) | None reported | Postexposure prophylaxis | 250 units in one dose of TIG | Used in conjunction with tetanus toxoid |
| Varicella | Possible increase in severe varicella pneumonia | Can cause congenital varicella with increased mortality in neonatal period; very rarely causes congenital defects | Varicella-zoster immune globulin (VZIG) | None reported | Not routinely indicated in healthy pregnant women exposed to varicella | 1 vial/kg in one dose of VZIG, up to 5 vials | Only indicated for newborns of mothers who developed varicella within 4 days prior to delivery or 2 days following delivery. Approximately 90–95% of adults are immune to varicella. |
| | | | *INACTIVATED VIRUS VACCINES* | | | | |
| Influenza | Possible increase in morbidity and mortality during epidemic of new antigenic strain | Possible increased abortion rate; no malformations confirmed | Inactivated type A and type B virus vaccines | None confirmed | Usually recommended only for patients with serious underlying diseases; public health authorities to be consulted for current recommendation | Consult with public health authorities since recommendations change each year | Criteria for vaccination of pregnant women same as for all adults |

## IMMUNIZATION DURING PREGNANCY *(Continued)*

| IMMUNIZING AGENT | RISK FROM DISEASE TO PREGNANT FEMALE | RISK FROM DISEASE TO FETUS OR NEONATE | TYPE OF IMMUNIZING AGENT | RISK FROM IMMUNIZING AGENT TO FETUS | INDICATIONS FOR IMMUNIZATION DURING PREGNANCY | DOSE SCHEDULE | COMMENTS |
|---|---|---|---|---|---|---|---|
| Rabies | Near 100% fatality; not altered by pregnancy | Determined by maternal disease | Killed virus vaccine | Unknown | Indications for prophylaxis not altered by pregnancy; each case considered individually | Public health authorities to be consulted for indications and dosage | |
| *INACTIVATED BACTERIAL VACCINES* | | | | | | | |
| Cholera | Significant morbidity and mortality; more severe during 3rd trimester | Increased risk of fetal death during 3rd trimester maternal illness | Killed bacterial vaccine | Unknown | Only to meet international travel requirements | 2 injections, 4–8 weeks apart | Vaccine of low efficacy |
| Meningococcus | No increased risk during pregnancy; no increase in severity of disease | Unknown | Killed bacterial vaccine | No data available on use during pregnancy | Indications not altered by pregnancy; vaccination recommended only in unusual outbreak situations | Public health authorities to be consulted | |

| | | | | | | |
|---|---|---|---|---|---|---|
| Plague | Significant morbidity and mortality; not altered by pregnancy | Determined by maternal disease | Killed bacterial vaccine | None reported | Very selective vaccination of exposed persons | Public health authorities to be consulted for indications and dosage |
| Pneumococcus | No increased risk during pregnancy; no increase in severity of disease | Unknown | Polyvalent polysaccharide vaccine | No data available on use during pregnancy | Indications not altered by pregnancy; vaccine used only for high-risk individuals | In adults 1 dose only |
| Typhoid | Significant morbidity and mortality; not altered by pregnancy | Unknown | Killed bacterial vaccine | None confirmed | Not recommended routinely except for close, continued exposure or travel to endemic areas | *Primary:* 2 injections, 4 weeks apart; *Booster:* single dose |

Source: American College of Obstetricians and Gynecologists. *Immunization During Pregnancy,*

ACOG Technical Bulletin 64. Washington, D.C.: ACOG, May

the United States), or hepatitis B are endemic may need vaccination.

    ° Most primelife mothers are already immune to measles, mumps, tetanus, typhoid, German measles (rubella), and diphtheria. This has mostly been accomplished by prior vaccinations, which incidentally need to be reinforced every ten years or so with but few exceptions.

    ° Rubella (German measles) is a minor viral disease that can have disastrous pregnancy effects and which by now should have disappeared from the United States. Unfortunately, because of our own neglect it has not disappeared and is even making a comeback. Rubella vaccine is safe and generally will produce lifetime immunity. It should not be given during pregnancy and, although often recommended, probably should not be given after delivery if nursing is contemplated.

    ° Hopefully no primelife mother will sustain a bite from a rabid animal. But sad to say, rabies is increasing rapidly in the animal population in this country. Thus, skunks, bats, raccoons, squirrels, chipmunks, possums, cattle, fox, and horses as well as dogs and cats are all vectors of rabies. The new human rabies vaccine is safe and easy to give. The human rabies immune globulin should be given as well as an initial treatment. Regardless of the potential fetal effects during pregnancy, both agents should be given to a primelife mother who has had a proven exposure to rabies.

    ° Hepatitis B is a very common form of liver disease in this country. It can cause untold damage to the child of an infected mother. There is a vaccine available now that can protect women vulnerable to hepatitis B infections—those living in endemic areas or who work in institutions for the mentally retarded, in hospital laboratories, or in operating rooms. Transmission to newborns can now be prevented by the vaccine in combination with hepatitis B immune globulin.

As a wrap-up, all immunization procedures that are contemplated for a primelife mother must be governed by the following considerations:

o Risk of exposure. If unavoidable circumstances expose a pregnant woman to an infectious hazard, then that fact must be weighed in the immunization decision—for example, a pregnant teacher during a flu epidemic.

o Risk from the disease. What effect will the disease, if contracted, have upon mother and babe? An example: rabies.

o Risks produced by the immunizing agent. Here must be determined the total risks to both mother and babe that the vaccinating agent may cause. Not a great deal is as yet known about some agents, but others are quite well studied. Rubella vaccine, for example, produces very specific fetal risks if given during pregnancy. Such risks are much less, however, than those produced by the actual disease itself. Thus abortion is no longer recommended for mothers who inadvertently receive the vaccine before they realize that they are pregnant. The Federal Center for Disease Control retains a hot line where you may obtain the very latest rubella information. The number is (404) 329-1862. Again, the rubella threat could be wiped away in one year by a national vaccination program. Betty Bumpers, wife of Senator Dale Bumpers (D-Arkansas), did just that in her home state. The last national rubella epidemic (1964–65) affected 30,000 pregnancies and cost the United States $1.5 billion. Think about that.

## IN AN EPIDEMIC

Most likely epidemics to occur in this country are outbreaks of influenza, measles (rubeola), or German measles (rubella), but no matter what the epidemic happens to be, you should:

o Consult your obstetrician before considering any vaccination. If you are in a foreign country, consult the American Embassy, the local WHO (World Health Organization) officer, the local public health officer, or call your obstetrician back home.

o Avoid public gatherings and close contact with other people. This would, alas, include your own family and children if they are attending school—a major source of infectious spread.

○ Most infections are droplet and hand transmitted—but mainly hand transmitted. Therefore, don't touch others and don't let their hands touch you. Don't use railings, push elevator buttons, or use doorknobs unless unavoidable. Wave, don't shake hands. Don't handle money!

○ Get plenty of rest and eat at home, rinsing and/or cooking food well.

## TRAVELING

We are a mobile society and most primelife mothers are probably on-the-go people. Even if you are not a traveler and cherish being a homeperson, you probably will get invited on some sort of fabulous trip while you are pregnant and simply have to go. Travel, however exciting or boring, always brings some kinds of problems—lost baggage, missed connections, language barriers, jet lag—or, closer to home, bad reservations, auto clinkers, detours, and so on. Now add to that swollen legs, fidget foot, nausea at the turn of a corner, midget bladder, and johns that are too small or too dirty and you have some grasp of what pregnant and footloose can mean.

Here are some basic travel suggestions for going anywhere on earth:

○ Don't travel far from home in the first trimester. Most abortions occur at this time. Likewise, avoid distant travel during the last month of even the most normal pregnancy since labor may easily begin during this time. Travel does not ordinarily induce abortions or premature labor, but being away from home at these times can be unpleasant if either event comes upon you.

○ You should be able to travel within a fifty- to one hundred-mile radius of your home at almost any time during pregnancy.

○ Always wear a seat belt in a car or an airplane and wear it all the time. It may cause some damage to you or to your baby in the event of an accident but the damage will be much less if you are belted in. This is an absolute, not a theory.

○ Be wary of sudden altitude changes. Cabin pressure in a commercial airline is the same as found at 7000 feet above sea level. Since you are not physically active on an airplane, there is no risk to you or your little one. In fact, commercial flying—if you keep your seat belt fastened at all times—is the safest way for you to travel. But if you are flying, say, from New York to Aspen, Colorado, to ski, you have about an 8000-foot altitude difference at Aspen Village from New York City and up to a 12,000-foot difference at the top of Big Burn. And while skiing you will be exerting yourself physically, sometimes maximally. This can have very harmful effects on both of you. Best you should acclimatize yourself over a forty-eight-hour period before hitting the slopes. Or perhaps ski in Vermont, which starts off closer to sea level.

○ While on the subject of flying, jet lag has no known harmful effect on pregnancy. It is, however, harder for a pregnant traveler to sustain. Eat lightly on the plane and don't drink alcohol. Drink extra fluids copiously, though, because you lose fluids very rapidly in the dry cabin environment. Plan to give your circadian cycle a good twenty-four hours to catch up with you at your destination. The x-ray devices at airports are said to be absolutely safe so far as fetal exposure is concerned.

○ Traveling by ship seems to be the most luxurious way to go. They always picture smiling chefs with a bountiful smorgasbord spread before them heaped with delicacies, festooned with glorious bottles of wine, all waiting just for you. Beware! The food may be older than the wine and may leave your stomach a lot faster! Ships have real problems in preserving food safely and even the venerable stars of the passenger lines have been known to fail American food inspector tests from time to time. So you might have your travel agent provide you with the latest USPHS inspection of your ship-to-be. Your agent has or can easily get that information. Eat lightly—a thing that cruise ships discourage—but go easy and remember that your digestion under the best of circumstances is not up to par just now.

○ Although your private, personal early pregnancy nausea may be long gone, seasickness may bring it home again temporarily. There is little you can take in the way of medication, so try and keep your fluid and sugar levels up through the crisis by way of soft drinks or clear soups.

o Traveler's diarrhea—hereinafter referred to as TD—affects 30 to 50 percent of all travelers, depending upon where they go. High-risk countries are found in Latin America, Africa, the Middle East, and Asia. Intermediate-risk destinations include Southern Europe and some Caribbean islands. Low-risk countries include the remaining Caribbeans (it varies), Canada, northern Europe, Australia, New Zealand, and the good ole USA.

TD is caused by the fecal contamination of food. After you digest that nauseous fact, you can understand the numerous dietary restrictions recommended by health officials. Avoid raw vegetables, meats, and seafood; tap water; ice; unpasteurized milk and dairy products; unpeeled fruits; and any incompletely cooked foods. On the other hand, carbonated beverages, beer, wine, hot coffee and tea, and properly bottled or boiled water are all safe. Avoid street vendors like the plague—they may be! At some hotels the ice is safely prepared and they usually make a point of advertising that fact.

TD usually lasts about four days. Any diarrhea lasting longer than that, or accompanied by fever or bloody bowel movements, needs immediate and competent medical management. Pepto-Bismol should accompany all travelers to risk areas. It is safe and effective for most simple TD. There is another antidiarrheal medicine available by prescription that is more effective than Pepto-Bismol called loperamide (Imodium). Its safety during pregnancy has not been established. So it's back to square one. Fluids need to be replaced along with glucose and electrolytes. Gatorade or the equivalent is an excellent source of replacement. Pregnant women should not take antibiotics as a prophylactic against TD. Some antibiotics have serious fetal effects. (See page 67.)

o Be sure your immunizations are current for the countries you are entering. Smallpox vaccination is no longer necessary anywhere, but diphtheria, tetanus, typhoid, and certain others will be necessary in some areas. (See Immunization, pages 72–81.) And be sure and consult your travel agent. If you can't communicate in the language of the countries you intend to visit, get a translator's dictionary that includes basic medical terms.

Here is a listing of some agencies that might help you when you are out in the world:

○ Airtransport Association of America, 1709 New York Avenue, Washington, D.C. 20006.

○ National Association of Truck Stop Operators, P.O. Box 1285, Alexandria, Virginia 22313. Telephone (703) 549-2100. They list truck stops that supply you with twenty-four-hour services of all kinds—sleep, laundry, food, bank, post office, etc.

○ Association for Medical Assistance to Travelers, Empire State Building, 350 Fifth Avenue, New York, New York 10001. For finding an English-speaking doctor in a foreign country.

○ The embassy of the United States of America no matter where you are outside of our boundaries.


## NUISANCES

Little things mean a lot, particularly when they are harmless little things, which, like a mosquito bite, don't alter the course of the world but which can make a primelife pregnancy or any pregnancy just a little more testy. Here are some of them. Harmless or not, these little demons of pregnancy can bug you outrageously.

### Leg cramps

Often, in the still of the night and in the last trimester of your pregnancy, you may awaken abruptly because one of your calf muscles is in such intense spasm that you could pole-vault out of the window on it if it weren't so painful. The ultimate cause of these leg cramps is not clearly decided by the experts, but I can tell you how to prevent them.

Well, if you are having one right now, get out of bed and stand on the afflicted leg, massage it, and if it doesn't shortly ease away, get into a warm tub bath. Of course, by the time the tub is drawn and ready for you, the cramp will surely be gone. The best course of action is prevention.

     ° If you are drinking milk, stop. Except for infants and starving populations, milk is not good food. (See pages 50–51.)

     ° Get supplements of calcium carbonate. Although most prenatal tablets contain calcium, you generally do not get enough in a one-a-day formula. There are many calcium carbonate tablets on the market and it doesn't matter if they are made from oyster shells or from the White Cliffs of Dover— calcium carbonate is calcium carbonate. Fifteen hundred milligrams a day will stop your leg cramps. Calcium is somewhat constipating so watch out. You don't want to replace your leg cramps with hemorrhoids.

## Heartburn

This little nuisance also develops in the last trimester—usually. Your beloved infant has now commandeered the vast majority of your abdomen, leaving the regular occupants little or no place to go. Thus, your stomach tries to move up into your chest—a move that is stoutly resisted by your heart and lungs. Nevertheless, the stomach wins and part of it will herniate—or move—into the chest and you have a diaphragmatic hernia—and heartburn. Further grief is encountered because the stomach fails to empty itself with the usual old dispatch, and so food and acid tend to accumulate therein. Your gastric problem is temporary. Help it by:

     ° Avoiding seasoned food, particularly pepper seasoning. Also, shy away from fatty foods and rich desserts.

     ° Don't eat before you lie down—or don't lie down after you eat. Either one.

     ° Some antacids are fine for you, but some are not. Ask your doctor.

     ° Cracked ice gives immediate, temporary, safe relief. You can chew it ad infinitum. It does pile up in the bladder, however, and that makes for another problem.

     ° During the night, it may be more comfortable to sleep—or try to sleep—somewhat propped up on pillows.

This position may help your stomach to empty. It's worth a try.

Heartburn will leave you the day you deliver—almost without exception.

## The carpal tunnel

There is a fibrous sheath called the carpal tunnel that encloses nerves and tendons leading into each hand. This sheath may swell with fluid—just as your hands and legs may—while pregnancy advances. If the carpal tunnel swells, your fingers may at first tingle and later feel numb—a most uncomfortable sensation. Besides elevating your arms above your head while reclining, there is little to do about this condition except to wait for delivery to whisk it away—which it will. Sometimes the same symptoms are produced by the thoracic outlet syndrome. This condition arises from pressure on the nerves as they leave your shoulders. Only special studies can determine which certain exercises are necessary to control the thoracic outlet problem. Such exercises have no effect on carpal tunnel problems.

## Stuffy ears and nose

The veins which drain blood away from the ears, the sinuses, and the nose generally dilate under the influence of pregnancy hormones. In fact, all your veins do that and you can see it happening to skin veins all over your body. At any rate, in the nose and ear area, such venous congestion produces nasal stuffiness and may make your ears feel like you have been flying in a plane. Again, this little nuisance must simply be tolerated. Do not try to use decongestants.

## Unstable joints

Relaxin is the name given to a hormone that floods the pregnant body. It comes from the pituitary gland, but it goes everywhere. Its avowed purpose is to relax the ligaments which hold the pelvic cavity together and which allows women—all of us—to walk upright. Such relaxation is supposed to facilitate labor and delivery by increasing joint mobility and give, and it does that. It also makes you fall on your face when the relaxation is too abundant. Your pelvic joints—particularly the hip joints—become very unstable and you must be careful in moving about or you really will fall because of the unstable joint mechanism.

Relaxin will sometimes make your pubic bones separate so much that their midline joint becomes very tender, both to touch and on movement. Very rarely will these bones separate completely—I have seen it only once. When it happens, bed rest is mandatory. Fortunately, the joint heals almost immediately after delivery.

## Umbilical hernia

You will see when your baby is born that the umbilical cord enters its body through the umbilicus, which, shortly after birth, seals over completely and becomes the belly button. Every once in a while, a small opening persists in this area, which almost never causes any problems. During some pregnancies, however, this small opening may get bigger and abdominal contents may herniate through it, causing an umbilical hernia. Although often uncomfortable and accompanied by an unsightly umbilical bulge, such hernias seldom require treatment and disappear at birth. Very rarely they will strangulate, cause acute pain, and require surgical intervention.

## Backache

Our sacroiliac joints, joints where the lower back and the hips meet one another, are often the target of strains and pains. This is particularly so during pregnancy because of the shift in body mechanics that accompanies a growing abdomen. Everything is pulled forward and pulled down, and so to compensate, the shoulders and upper spine must be tilted back, thus causing a shearing effect on the sacroiliac area. To see this clearly, look at the profile of a standing full-term pregnant woman and you will see how far back she must lean to keep from falling forward. You can get the same picture looking at the standing profile of any man with a big enough paunch to require his belt to hang below it and still by some kind of magic hold his pants up.

After delivery the tone of all abdominal muscles has been badly undone—as you will give testimony to when your feet first hit the floor and your supposedly empty abdomen has not changed in any way that you can perceive. Thus, there is a tendency to keep the exaggerated pelvic tilt of pregnancy and so the sacroiliac grind will continue and so will backache. What to do?

**PREVENTION**

      o Practice postural exercises and pregnancy-safe aerobic exercises.

      o Sleep on a firm mattress or water bed and lie on your side with your knees pulled up as tight as you can as often as you can.

      o Avoid physical activity or sports that could further strain an already strained back. Your common sense will tell you what these activities are.

      o Avoid high heels.

      o Control your weight gain.

      o Exercise, exercise, exercise—but sensibly.

**MANAGEMENT**

      o A girdle may be necessary to help support your back. Once a common part of women's armamentarium, girdles have fallen into dissuse lately for a number of reasons—one of them being that they give artificial support and muscles come to depend upon this external support rather than going to work themselves. But, anyway, you may need one, at least temporarily, to prevent increasing damage to your back.

      o As in prevention, sleeping or resting on your side with knees drawn up tight will help relieve the pelvic crunch.

      o A good massage and local heat will help and will certainly make you feel better, particularly if tenderly done by a very close, deeply involved co-impregnator.

      o Complete bed rest with medications rarely may be necessary. All this is under the jurisdiction of your own doctor.

      o Exercise, exercise, exercise—when it's safe. Follow earlier guidelines found on pages 34–41.

## Rib pain

Again, let me say that your growing baby is trying to push everything that is in your stomach into your chest. Since that doesn't work, several alternates come into play. One of these alternates is the expansion of your rib cage, which may lead to the spontaneous separation of a few of your lower ribs, particularly those on your right side. Usually this event takes place in the last trimester, and as any speared quarterback can tell you, rib separation is not a very pleasant experience. You will notice discomfort over the separated lower ribs when you breathe deeply, or when you are hugged, or just when you move around. There is nothing to do about it, no harm from it, and like everything else, it will go away delivery day. Hallelujah!!

## SKIN

The hide that binds is subject to a considerable mauling as pregnancy inflates it. It is stretched in many ways and in many places. The growing uterus stretches abdominal skin, growing breasts stretch their skin, widening bone structure stretches the flank skin, and finally, edema stretches arm and leg skin. Not much is left unstretched. The hormones related to pregnancy also exert powerful influences on the skin, and in a variety of ways. Certain skin diseases occur only during pregnancy and sometimes represent real hazards to the continuing health of that pregnancy.

### Stretching

○ Stria. Skin, particularly thin skin, will, when stretched, tear—not split open, but tear in its underlying supportive layers. As a result, linear red streaks begin to appear over the abdomen, breasts, and thighs. These lines are called stria (plural, striae) and alas, though they fade to silver after delivery, they never completely disappear. Regular massaging with lanolin-based skin creams helps minimize the striae.

○ Pain and no pain. Stretching the skin also stretches the tiny cutaneous nerve endings that underlie it. As a result of this, areas of skin on the upper abdomen become painful to touch. Eventually, these areas become numb and remain so for the rest of the pregnancy. Such painful or numb spots may occur anywhere on the body where there has been enough skin spread.

## Hormones

o Dilated veins. First over the breasts and then generally, superficial veins become dilated. They become very easy to trace as they course through the deeper skin layers. Although they may appear ugly to you, they are not and anyway, they cannot be altered. In susceptible individuals, dilation of the leg veins may help increase the tendency toward varicose veins. In this situation, support pantyhose will be of great value.

o Zits. Women who have suffered from acne for years may find that pregnancy banishes it completely. On the other hand, women with glorious complexions may suddenly find themselves laden with adolescent zits once again. There is no way of telling how any individual skin will react and neither extreme may be noted, but both the afflicted and the un-afflicted skin revert back to their original state after pregnancy is done with. Special acne care may be needed for some of these skins.

o Cherry spots. Often very tiny red bumps that are not the least bit tender, inflamed, or irritated appear on the chest and arms. Only a few of these little cherry bumps appear and they usually go away within a few months after delivery.

o Chloasma. This mottled darkening of the skin is generally confined to the face alone and it is made much worse by sunlight. Often the forehead, the bridge of the nose, and cheeks are most afflicted, but one nonface area, the areola around each breast, commonly darkens too. Nothing can be done except with makeup. Avoid sunlight or tanning booths since this accentuates the darkening. Chloasma gradually fades after delivery, but the darkened breast areola never fades.

## Skin disorders

○ Iron, such as that found in prenatal supplements, can produce a red rash over the torso which oftentimes is itchy and irritating. Should iron be the suspected culprit, proof can easily be obtained by stopping the supplement. Within a few days all will be clear again and another source of iron must be found.

○ Herpes gestationis. There is no relationship between this skin disorder and the herpes that has us all on our ears. Only the name is the same. Herpes gestationis is characterized by an itchy eruption over most of the body which generally begins after midpregnancy and may even begin after delivery. It simply has to run its course—there is no known cause or cure. It can, in some way also unknown, have a damaging effect on pregnancy. Fortunately, it is rare.

○ Pruritis gravidarum. This consists of generalized itching without any skin eruption to accompany it. Usually it occurs in the last months and goes away without a trace or without any harm—unless it's from scratching.

○ Pruritic urticaria of pregnancy. These benign urticarial lesions occur in about 1 of every 250 pregnancies and are slightly more common in the primelife. Generally very itchy, they first appear on the lower abdomen and thighs, spreading to the trunk and upper arms. This skin disease of unknown cause generally appears in the third trimester and disappears within a week after delivery. There are no harmful effects upon mother or child, and only topical treatment is used.

So, with all this surface tension in mind, you need to take special care of your primelife skin. Avoid heavy makeup and avoid much sunlight and/or tanning equipment. Keep your skin well oiled and supported when and where necessary. Remember, excess weight gain means more skin stretching and more lines, and afterward, more wrinkles. Beauty may not be only skin deep—but it starts there.

## PERSPIRATION

Sweat glands are located in the deeper skin layers and sweat appears first on the skin before it gets on everything else, and so it is logical to talk about it here.

Sweating helps regulate body temperature, which is elevated in pregnancy. Sweat also exudes certain characteristic odors. A marked increase in sweating is not uncommon during pregnancy, and this may be a source of some discomfort and displeasure—except to your laundryperson. Moreover, changes in your skin metabolism may invite a different type of skin bacteria to take up residence, which may alter the odor upon your body. These undesireable changes cannot be driven away during pregnancy and only frequent showers and antiperspirants or deodorants—or both—will keep you feeling as you want.

## HEADACHES

Each year, about 80 percent of us succumb to headaches of some sort. No wonder so much advertising money is spent on this affliction. There are three main headache types: tension (50 percent); migraine (20 percent); neurological (30 percent). Any of them may—and do—occur in pregnancy and while migraine seems to ease at that time, tension headaches tend to increase. No treatment other than acetaminophen (Tylenol, etc.) may be taken while pregnant, unless ordered by your obstetrician.

Pregnancy seems to produce a particular little headache all of its own. This headache—often overlooked in the textbooks—generally makes its appearance early on and disappears sometime in the second trimester. It is a dull frontal headache that tends to ease away during periods of rest and sleep. The cause is not clearly known, but it is believed related to the instability of blood pressure that begins in early pregnancy and that also causes drowsiness and syncope. Philosophically, it is easier to bear this nuisance knowing that it is limited by time.

Should hypertension of pregnancy occur during the last trimester, a different type of headache may accompany it. This is a neurological headache, caused by swelling of the brain tissues and by hypertension. It is usually a generalized headache often accompanied by blurred vision or other visual disturbances. It should be reported to your doctor immediately.

## BREASTS

According to anatomists, the female mammary gland is a somewhat conical mass of glandular tissue transversed and supported by strands of fibrous tissue and covered by a thick layer of fat. And each breast lies on the anterior thorax, usually between the fourth and ninth rib. According to the centerfold and stapling industry, the female mammary gland is something entirely else. The erotic interest generated by the female breasts in our society has defied logical explanation by our scientific community—no matter how many government grants have been fed to it or how many scientists have been engrossed in it. For our primelife purposes, you and I will play it straight. Here are some breast changes that you will notice:

° Early engorgement. Very shortly after conception your breasts become congested, firm, and tender. Looking in the mirror, you may be able to see bluish veins coursing just under the skin of each breast. All these are normal changes that gradually abate in the early months only to reappear later. A thin, watery discharge may now appear at the nipples, particularly during breast stimulation. This fluid is colostrum, a forerunner of milk, and this nipple drainage continues off and on during pregnancy. Unless you have to prove some kind of point, you will be more comfortable with some breast support, and if much troubled with colostrum, may want to wear a nursing shield.

° Breast growth. After the initial surge of congestion, your breasts soften, but continue to grow somewhat as pregnancy advances. Further, the pinkish area around each nipple, the areola, tends to become darker brown, the latter generally causing more concern than the former. Anyway, that's the way it is.

° Striae. As the breasts grow, they stretch the skin that attempts to contain them. Such stretching often causes reddish furrows or lines to form in the skin and these are called striae. Such lines may also appear on the abdomen and thighs as well. Regular massage with a lanolin-based skin cream helps a great deal and there should be eager help available for this task at all times and for all anatomical sites.

o Nipples. Usually the nipples become darker as times goes on and become more prominently everted. Should you have nipple inversion so that they are not clearly visible, it is important—if you are planning to nurse—that this situation be corrected. Each night when you are massaging your breasts (or they are being massaged) the nipples should be stripped outward gently till they eventually stay out. Even if this cannot be accomplished completely by delivery time, it still helps and a nursing shield will help further when nursing is established.

Important note: If you have a history of premature labor or any tendency toward it in this pregnancy, do not massage your nipples *for any reason* or engage in breast foreplay during love-making. (See page 269.)

## VAGINAL INFECTIONS

Vaginal secretions are normally somewhat acid and are made up of:

o Mucous secreted by the cervix.

o A clear liquid transudate that regularly weeps across the vaginal lining.

o Superficial skin cells that exfoliate (break away) by the billions from the constantly growing vaginal epithelium (skin).

o Bacteria which normally colonize the vagina and are necessary for vaginal hygiene and health.

o Lactic acid. Normal vaginal epithelium cells are rich in glycogen (sugar). Bacteria break glycogen down into lactic acid and thus add the characteristic odor to vaginal secretions.

Normal healthy vaginal secretions are increased during pregnancy because of the intense local congestion that occurs. Thus, a heavier discharge is not unusual, but its characteristics should be unchanged. Should the secretions become irritating, offensive, painful, or bloody, you need help.

There are two relatively minor vaginal infections to contend with during pregnancy—yeast and trichomonas.

## Yeast

This is the most common vaginal infection of all—and one of the most irritating. Generally there is redness and swelling at the vagina entrance and a thick white discharge. If, for some important reason, you need an antibiotic while you are pregnant, you become much more susceptible to a vaginal yeast infection, and probably should be prepared for it. Suppositories and creams are available which are quite effective, but which cannot prevent a recurrence. Yeast infections can be—and often are—sexually transmitted from your partner's penis, hands, or mouth. However, it is not a venereal disease because the organisms are everywhere—even on your own body—although you are usually resistant to them. To protect yourself from reinfection from any source put paper around all toilet seats; shower, don't tub bathe; wear a panty liner and avoid sex until all symptoms subside.

To douche or not to douche? Douching is a personal form of cleansing hygiene that women resorted to many centuries before the word was invented. Like gargling, tooth care, soap, perfume, and eyeliner, it has been a woman's device to attain the degree of personal fastidiousness and charm that suited her best interests.

Today most douches consist of disposable syringe equipment and are loaded with a variety of pleasing chemicals that may produce a local euphoria, but that may also be a source of irritation and allergy. Prepackaged vinegar and water douches are the least likely to irritate and generally the safest to use.

Pregnancy alters douching customs somewhat in that the cervix becomes soft and may be entered accidentally by the douching nozzle. Thus, douche liquids may directly enter the uterus, with very bad consequences. For this reason, most obstetricians—male and female alike—advise against douching during pregnancy. Thus, if douching is part of your regular armamentarium, you need to check with your own doctor first.

But to return to yeast infections—although douching with

disposable vinegar and water equipment is cleansing and comforting at other times, you must avoid it while pregnant, unless your own obstetrician recommends it.

## Trichomonas

This mild sexually transmitted (usually) vaginal infection is caused by a single-cell organism that dwells in and around the vagina and in and around the male prostate gland. When the vagina is involved there is usually a thin yellow discharge of unpleasant odor and there is also usually itching and irritation inside and out. The infection readily responds in most cases to a chemical agent called metronidazole, which is taken by mouth and which of course cannot be given during pregnancy. There are certain vaginal suppositories which are of help as are vinegar douches if allowed. Moreover, the preventive hygiene described above for yeast infections should be followed with this infection as well. Trichomonas infections have no known effect on pregnancy. Apparently its most serious side effect is upon interpersonal relationships: Who brought it home?

## Bacterial vaginosis (BV)

This is a relatively new term coined for a relatively old bacterial infection of the vagina. Previous names include hemophilus vaginitis, and Gardnerella vaginitis. No matter—the infection is bacterial, very common, and accompanied by a malodorous fishy odor. It is very difficult to diagnose accurately, very common, and usually responds to metronidazole as does trichomonas. So it cannot be treated during pregnancy either. This infection may— just may—have a role in premature rupture of the membranes in late pregnancy or in small-for-dates pregnancies, and that is why I hesitated to include it in minor pregnancy vaginal infections. This inferred role is still not proven, but it makes sense to eliminate such infections before a planned pregnancy.

Some serious vaginal infections may complicate pregnancy. Such infections are considered serious because they can damage a fetus as well as its host. All of these are sexually transmitted— some bacterial, some viruses.

## Chlamydia

A bacterial infection, this particular STD (sexually transmitted disease) is probably number one on the STD list today, although others keep crowding it. The symptoms are only a mildly irritating, usually yellowish discharge. Often the discharge goes unnoticed and, in the nonpregnant state, can silently produce tubal closure and thus sterility. Chlamydia is implicated in premature rupture of the membranes, premature labor, and even SIDS. Two thirds of the babies born to infected mothers will contract the infection during vaginal delivery.

Tests are fortunately now available for chlamydia, thus making the diagnosis easier in suspected cases. Tetracycline, the most effective treatment, cannot be used during pregnancy. Erythromycin is generally substituted. Barrier contraceptives offer significant protection at all times.

## Gonorrhea

Once a popular pelvic passenger, this bacteria-caused STD is losing ground to the newer infections. Yes, it is still increasing—particularly newer, more resistant, mutant forms—but it is not increasing as fast as its running mates. The discharge from gonorrhea is usually heavy, yellow, and irritating. It can be cultured easily and treated with appropriate penicillins—to which, as mentioned, it becomes more resistant all the time. Penicillin can be used during pregnancy. Infants delivered vaginally in the presence of gonorrhea risk permanent blindness if not treated at once. Many states have laws that provide for immediate treatment of all newborns' eyes. The rationale behind such laws is fast fading—and so are the laws. But when gonorrhea is present, eye treatment is mandatory.

## Mycoplasmosis

This is a less common member of the STD cult and is virtually symptom-free. It is usually discovered in an infertility work-up by blood testing since it is virtually impossible to culture in most clinical settings. Besides infertility its main effect on pregnancy is its involvement in repeated spontaneous abortions. Treatment is with specific antibiotics and the results may be followed by regular blood testing.

### Beta hemolytic streptococcus

This is a fairly common disease-causing bacteria found in many other parts of the body. Whether it is sexually transmitted or not is still unsettled, but it probably is. Beta strep can be found in 2 percent of all vaginal cultures, and it is implicated as one of the causative agents in premature rupture of the membranes. Very little discharge—or none at all—is related to this organism's presence in the vagina. It cultures easily and responds to penicillin therapy. Since its role is not yet clearly defined, some obstetricians routinely culture for it, some do not.

There appear to be no simple, harmless viral infections of the vagina, and as newer forms evolve they seem to become more violent in their effect. For example, AIDS, which can start as a vaginal infection and is, of course, a virus, will sooner or later destroy its host. (See pages 236–37.) Most viral vaginal infections are not, thank God, so vicious.

### Condyloma

This is the name given to warts found in the vagina and vulva in ever greater numbers in recent years. They are caused by the human papilloma virus. Such sexually transmitted warts are very difficult to eradicate, and if present at or near the time of birth, may cause papillomas of the fetal larynx any time up to five years later but usually during the first year. They often grow rapidly during pregnancy and are very often associated with premalignant changes in the cervix, which may have to be treated no matter what the duration of pregnancy. Treatment involves prolonged local applications, even laser surgery. Since it is an STD, reinfection is common even if the male consort has no visible lesions.

### Herpes virus II

Until recently, herpes virus II has led the hit parade for sensational journalism. The disease has not changed in any way, but the

sensationalists have moved on to the greener pastures of chlamydia and AIDS. There are obviously at least two kinds of herpes.
Number I has been responsible for cold sores that for generations
have appeared from time to time around the mouth of susceptible
individuals. Herpes II, on the other hand, is an STD with many
thousands of variations and virulences that has recently taken up
residence in American genitals, and since oral/genital sex has
replaced baseball as the national pastime, both herpes I and II can
be found in oral or genital locations. Only cultures—difficult to
obtain—can differentiate one from the other. Blood tests can tell
if infection has taken place, but such tests cannot tell when or
where the infections started. So we get into a very real and deep
social, moral, philosophical, and medical web when such ulcers
are found. Who brought them home? Usually, the ulcers are no-
ticed around the vaginal or rectal entrance, are about one quarter
inch across, shallow, and very painful at least for the first week.
After that, they gradually heal and disappear only to burst forth
at regular intervals thereafter. There are local treatments that are
safe during pregnancy, but oral systemic medicines must be avoided.

Herpes' effects upon pregnancy include:

- Early abortion.
- Premature labor.
- Transmission to the baby at delivery.
- A disseminated maternal infection.

How frequent a problem is herpes in pregnancy? Well, about
1 percent of all pregnant women have genital herpes—that would
come to 37,000 deliveries annually. Yet, of these, only 400 cases
of neonatal herpes are reported each year. These cases are, however, usually devastating and are accompanied by a 70 percent
fetal mortality rate.

How to manage:

- Give your obstetrician any history of previous herpes
lesions.

- Immediately report any signs of herpes recurrence during pregnancy.

○ Make sure your doctor takes appropriate cultures, smears, or blood tests as indicated.

○ Vaginal delivery will be undertaken if repeated and recent cultures are negative and no lesions are noted by the mother and none seen by the obstetrician at the beginning of labor. Otherwise a cesarian section is the preferred method of delivery even though it does not represent a perfect preventative for the newborn.

○ After delivery, mother should wash her hands thoroughly before handling her baby. Herpes is not transmitted by breast milk and so nursing, in the light of present knowledge, is safe. If an oral herpes lesion is present on mother, she should wear a mask while feeding and handling her baby.

## BOWEL MANAGEMENT DURING PREGNANCY

If you have been accustomed to problem-free bowels and regular elimination in the past, you may have to accept some adjustments during pregnancy. If, on the other hand, you have already suffered some bowel disturbances, particularly constipation, you may find the situation worsening as pregnancy advances. There are several reasons for this:

○ Bowel tone decreases.

○ Fluid balance is altered and less fluid accumulates in the intestinal tract. Although it often doesn't feel like it, stools are 90 percent water!

○ Mechanical pressure caused by a growing baby and local pelvic congestion tend to produce a feeling of fullness and further increases the possibility of hemorrhoids (piles).

Regular soft bowel movements should be your goal. This is best achieved by:

○ Establishing a regular time to eliminate—and responding to it—regardless. At any other time in the day it should also be answered at once, but in time the urge stabilizes.

○ Make a conscious effort to drink fluids all day long. Water is your best hydrator—coffee, tea, and alcohol, your worst.

○ Eat bulk. That doesn't mean packing chips, sawdust, newspaper, or cellophane (although these materials are present in some "foods" advertised as bulk). In the cereal group it means bran and whole wheat; in the vegetables, squash and related high-fiber plants, lettuce, spinach, and other leafy vegetables; in the fruits, apples, oranges, grapefruit, melons, and the like. Prunes (dried plums) are of course in a class by themselves!

In the event that all the above fails to produce regular activity the first step is to add more bulk in the form of fiber, Metamucil being but one example of many available bulk agents. Taken as instructed, these are safe, well-tolerated, and effective in what they do. If you still need a push, laxatives and/or enemas may be needed. For the correct procedure here, you should call your obstetrician.

Iron, which is present in almost all prenatal vitamin/mineral preparations, often increases the tendency to constipation. Stopping the pills for a week demonstrates that effect and in such a case some other method of iron administration must be found. Conversely, iron causes diarrhea in some individuals and here again it must be given in some other way once it has been demonstrated to be the culprit. While on the subject of iron, this important mineral taken orally can also produce a generalized irritating rash that disappears promptly when the iron pills are stopped. Finally, sometimes all the iron taken is not absorbed and it turns into black iron oxide while in the colon and thus bowel movements become black. To the unprepared this bathroom discovery can be alarming, particularly since a hemoccult colon cancer test will be positive because such tests react to iron. You can prove you're okay by stopping the iron for a week.

Chronic constipation or just chronic bearing down can force the rectal veins to dilate (internal hemorrhoids) and eventually come down outside the rectum (external hemorrhoids). Thus exposed, the veins can rupture and bleed, form painful clots, and cause pain and itching in a most inconvenient and inaccessible area. Such problems need professional care. Hemorrhoids are more common in pregnancy, as we have seen, because of local pressure and congestion. In order to prevent them you should:

- Follow the regular rules above.

- When you do have a bowel movement, do not strain down if you feel incompletely empty. Most likely you will then be trying to push out dilated rectal veins with all their subsequent problems. Relax, sit still for a moment, and the congested veins will decongest and that full feeling will subside.

Special preexisting bowel diseases that may complicate a primelife pregnancy are covered in chapter 7.

## LONG TIME NO Z'S

Sleep, which is a natural physiological function, which "knits up the ravell'd sleave of care" and is "the balm of hurt minds, great nature's second course," and "chief nourisher in life's feast," has become a precious commodity denied to more and more of us as times goes on. Thus, for whatever reason, one third of all adults admit to sleep problems and physicians write about 55,000 prescriptions for sleeping pills *each* and *every* day—or night. So insomnia is a major disorder of our civilization and a symptom that is being studied more deeply all the time. Sleep labs are popping up all over the country and treatment clinics are available in most large communities—where most insomnia is found.

Whatever your sleeping habits have been, pregnancy has a major impact upon them. And the impact begins almost as soon as the pregnancy does. Thus, in the days shortly following conception, it becomes evident that the mother-to-be is very sleepy most of the time. This somnolent state has been mentioned before as an early symptom of pregnancy and it will disappear as the middle months come along. Until it does, give in to it and sleep. Insomnia is rarely a complication of early pregnancy.

Later pregnancy is different. There are many things that will rob you of sleep in the later months such as:

- Increased body metabolism producing increased body heat and awareness.

○ Increased pressure from within the abdomen both above and below.

○ Frequent need to empty the bladder.

○ Fetal movement.

○ General discomfort and inability to find and stay in a comfortable sleeping position.

○ Regurgitation of stomach contents with heartburn.

○ Unpleasant dreams—see below.

○ A mate who snores.

This is a frightening and formidable list and you may not have to cope with all of the problems listed above. Nevertheless, sleep is a very precious commodity as term approaches and is, as you can see, beset by a number of blockades. Here are some helpful hints:

○ Go to bed to sleep. Don't read, rest, or watch TV in bed. If you have a medical problem requiring rest (e.g., hypertension), use a sofa or couch in another room, and avoid your bed if possible.

○ If you take a nap, be sure it is early in the day.

○ Eliminate background noise as much as possible or mask such noises with wash-out or white sound. Tapes of such sounds (rain, seashore, etc.) are available everywhere. Sometimes a room fan provides the desired effect and is soothing by itself.

○ Avoid caffeine substances after 4:00 P.M. and cut down on fluids before bedtime.

○ If you have heartburn and regurgitate, don't eat before bedtime, keep recommended antacids at hand, and try sleeping semipropped up. Cracked ice is a safe and unlimited but temporary (what isn't?) cure for heartburn. Unfortunately, it melts and eventually has to go somewhere and your bladder advises you of its accumulation.

○ A water bed or a foam rubber egg-crate–shaped mattress may provide you with more comfort.

○ Fantasize or focus on an interesting task or situation. In some instances, the reverse is true and focusing on a boring task (counting sheep) works better. Condition yourself to one or the other.

○ Have a very close friend give you a gentle massage.

Sleeping pills are generally not prescribed during pregnancy.

## To sleep, perchance to dream

Dreaming, which occurs during light sleep periods, is often greatly enhanced during pregnancy. There is more light sleep. Unpleasant dreams and nightmares are unfortunately also more common. Such dreams frequently center around bad pregnancy outcomes. It may be reassuring to you to know that these dreams, unfortunate and frightening though they may be, bear no relationship to the health or the outcome of pregnancy. There is no effective way to prevent these dreams. Sharing them with someone close often diminishes their impact and they will be gone when you deliver.

## ACCIDENTS

Heaven forbid that you should be involved in any kind of serious accident while you are pregnant, but almost 10 percent of you will, and the risk increases as pregnancy advances, over half of all accidents occurring in the last trimester. Since you are becoming increasingly unstable, minor falls are not uncommon. You already know about high heels and their avoidance after the early months. Still, tripping on stairs and around bathtubs is very common, so watch out.

Your instability also makes you less responsive while you are driving. You must wear your seat belt always and drive defensively. Automobile accidents are a leading cause of maternal— and, alas, fetal—death in some areas of the United States. A seat belt protects you both.

Whether your injury is sustained at work, at play, or in an auto, here is some data for you:

○ The fetus is protected very well from injury during the early months. After that, as the uterus rises in the abdomen, it is a far more available unprotected target for injury. Your seat belt, worn properly, causes significantly less damage than its avoidance.

○ Pregnancy alters your response to injury and often changes the usual signs and symptoms of an injury. Whoever attends you should be told you are pregnant, for this and many other reasons. You should also know and carry with you a record of your blood type. Rh negative mothers may need Rh immune globulin shortly after some types of accidents.

○ Get fetal monitoring or real-time ultrasound as soon as you can after injury. It is important and may be very reassuring. You should also monitor your baby's activity yourself for several days following any significant trauma. During those same days watch carefully for any vaginal bleeding or watery discharge and for any unusual abdominal tenderness.

○ If it is possible, lie on your left side rather than on your back while you are awaiting help or being transported. This gets more blood to your baby.

○ Have knowledge of the best trauma center in your area. If you are injured while traveling, be sure that you are taken to a trauma center if indeed one is available.

○ As a very dear person used to say to his Hill Street charges, "Hey, be careful out there."

○○○○○○○○○○○○○ **THINGS TO THINK ABOUT** ○○○○○○○○○○○○○

Have bugs, will travel. Tourists are forever carrying diseases back and forth across the oceans. For instance, when Hernando Cortes visited the New World some 400 years ago, he and his valiant 600 brought smallpox along with them. That monstrous virus quickly decimated 3 million Mexicans.

Similarly, a group of tourists visiting in and around Cuba returned to their Spanish home, bringing with them a sexually transmitted disease that swept through Europe and Asia, killing, in a few years' time, untold millions of people from castle to gutter and destroying—or maiming forever—untold millions of newborn infants. The disease ravaged on for centuries. Its name? Syphilis. The tourists? Columbus and his crew.

Recently some tourists from this side of the ocean returned

the favor, perhaps with a stopover in Haiti. They brought home to us AIDS which they found—somehow—in the African green monkey. AIDS threatens to decimate this country and to maim or destroy countless innocent babes, since mothers carrying the virus will almost surely give it to their intrauterine infants—just as surely as syphilis was transmitted to unborn infants centuries ago.

○ ○ ○ ○ ○ ○ ○

We obstetricians often fail to take advantage of our special patient (or client) relationship during pregnancy to stress the importance of seat belt protection. Buckling up is rapidly becoming the law of the land, and, while some of us look upon it as a further intrusion into our personal affairs, there is no doubt left that it is a wise habit to form. Here are the results of some recent studies:

○ Automobile accidents are the leading cause of nonobstetric death of pregnant women in the United States today.

○ Less than 20 percent of all pregnant women use their seat belts. In one recent study, only 4 out of 115 buckled up.

○ Repeated studies have shown that lap/shoulder restraints significantly reduce maternal and fetal automobile mortality.

○ To be effective, the seat belts must be worn properly—over the lap and not the abdomen.

○ Eighty-one percent of surveyed obstetricians regularly wear seat belts while driving. Fewer than one third advised their expectant mothers to harness in.

○ When automobile safety was included in prenatal classes, the use of child care safety increased from 60 to 94 percent.

○ ○ ○ ○ ○ ○ ○

Even staying in bed is not safe. Last year there were 200,000 injuries sustained in, on, or under that piece of furniture—a few of them water related! Of course, many other "accidents" that occurred in and around beds are now showing up at obstetricians' offices.

○ ○ ○ ○ ○ ○ ○ ○ ○ ○ ○ ○ ○ ○ ○ ○ ○ ○ ○ ○ ○ ○ ○ ○ ○ ○ ○ ○ ○ ○ ○ ○ ○ ○ ○ ○ ○ ○ ○ ○ ○ ○ ○

## Mother, fetus, and the law

Suppose:

○ A pregnant woman is in an automobile accident and her fetus is born with injuries sustained by the accident. Can it recover damages for its injuries? In all states it can if it lives. In about half of the states the parent(s) can recover damages if it is born dead.

○ The fetus is killed in an accident, but it is nonviable. Can the parents recover damages? No state allows recovery under such circumstances.

○ A pregnant woman is an alcoholic or a drug abuser or engages in other activities known to be harmful to her fetus. Can she be prosecuted? No. The courts currently hold that a mother cannot be held liable no matter how she abuses her unborn fetus. Certain already proposed, ambiguous laws designed to prevent elective induced abortions may inadvertently alter this situation.

○ A pregnant woman needs a blood transfusion to sustain her life and that of her fetus, but she refuses on moral or other grounds. Can she be forced to submit to a transfusion? Yes, almost without exception.

○ A cesarian section is necessary, in the opinion of the attending doctors, to save an infant's life. Can it be forced upon a mother against her will? Yes, insofar as present court tests have been settled.

The conflicts that arise in courts today relative to maternal-fetal interests really come down to two issues:

○ Can a pregnant woman be held responsible for actions that are potentially damaging to her fetus?

○ Can a pregnant woman be forced to accept treatment to which she objects because of fetal interests?

The situations posed above illustrate the present legal climate in which these conflicts live. Soon, new conflicts will arise and will beg the courts for legal positions. For example, as fetal surgery evolves, can a mother be forced into a surgical procedure in her uterus (and, therefore, her body) and accept the risks to herself in order to salvage her fetus? That's going to be a tough one.

These legal conflicts beg answers to questions that are almost beyond resolution. If the courts eventually agree that mothers must be quarantined in order to stop their smoking or drinking or whatever, how can this be enforced? If she refuses to accept prenatal care, how can that be enforced? If her doctors feel she needs a tertiary care center, but she wishes to deliver at home with a midwife, how can that be prevented?

The law and, therefore, society seem to be heartily concerned with punitive measures to penalize mothers who, according to our standards, have transgressed against their fetuses. In actual fact, we are indeed more interested in punishing than preventing—much like a parent who would rather whip a child for scribbling on the walls than provide it with a blackboard. If we (and, through us, the government) really care about the welfare of fetuses—and their mothers—we would:

- Provide universal access to adequate prenatal care.

- Provide food for expectant mothers.

- Work diligently to banish tobacco, alcohol, and drugs from America.

- Provide mothers with adequate leave of absence from work with guaranteed continuation of pension and seniority rights.

- Educate all our children so that they might avoid a teenage pregnancy.

- Provide access to adequate delivery services for all mothers.

# ∘ 4 ∘
# Getting Ready

## PREPARATION FOR CHILDBIRTH

In the good old days, preparation for childbirth consisted of getting together newspapers and whiskey—or a bullet—and, of course, boiling water. Today the resources available for parental and sibling education in childbearing are enormous, almost overwhelming. And it all apparently began with Dr. Grantly Dick-Read.

In the early 1950's Dr. Dick-Read published his still available book, *Childbirth Without Fear,* in which he held that much pain of labor and delivery was associated with fear, tension, apprehension, and ignorance of what was going on. He advised and taught understanding of the birth process, and associated exercises and drills to promote relaxation during labor and to dispel fear. His program was very well accepted and widely used. His principles have formed the basis of many other programs and are still in wide use.

Currently, the Lamaze approach to preparedness is in favor. Dr. Lamaze taught that women should be prepared both emotionally and psychologically for childbearing in accordance with Pavlov's theory of the conditioned response. This theory states that the brain can be trained to select its response to any given stimulus. Applied to the discomfort and pain attendant upon labor and delivery, training could shift the focus away to another positive response. Lamaze interpretations vary widely from country to country, from city to city, and indeed, from one part of the community to another.

No matter what preparedness classes offer for the management of discomforts associated with labor and delivery, they also incorporate educational material which helps to explain the unfolding of pregnancy as well as labor and delivery. Exercises of many kinds are also included in the curriculum and the programs are being expanded to include siblings, grandparents, and God knows who else—pets and neighbors before long. Good things have a way of getting out of hand.

Here are some points about classes:

○ Instruction should begin early in the third trimester, and classes are usually held at hospitals, large clinics, churches, or various service organization headquarters. Your doctor can help you find a suitable one for you. Your mate or a support person who will be with you in labor should come with you, but it is not obligatory.

○ Pain. Pain is a very personal thing. Interior linemen thrive on it as do writers who send unsolicited manuscripts to publishers. Most other people find pain a reminder that they are in some jeopardy and react by withdrawing from it. Even so, pain thresholds vary widely among all of us.

This is simply to point out that what may be a joyous painless experience to one mother may be a shattering nightmare to another, no matter how well and diligently prepared. Moreover, because of a variety of anatomical considerations, some labors are associated with a great deal more discomfort than others.

The bottom line: No matter how well-trained you may be, there may come a time in your labor—be it early or late—that you want some professional pain management. No amount of peer pressure or misguided coaching should make you feel guilty for accepting help at this time. You are not going to have to apologize to anyone for failing. If you do, you have been to the wrong classes. And you have failed nothing.

○ A great number of men enjoy coaching women through labor and watching the fruit of their love as it is being born. A number of men don't, and for them to participate in all this against their will, because of peer pressure or whatever, is not a rewarding or healthy experience. There is a growing body of evidence that such exposure can be psychologically devastating to some men and, further, can destroy the relationship it was meant to enhance. Let each one march to the beat of their own drummer. After all, family strength and bonds are considerably weaker today with all our togetherness than they were when delivery was a very private affair.

It is altogether advisable, then, to attend a reliable preparedness course that gives you meaningful education, insight into the labor and delivery phenomenon, a reasonable exercise program, no fantasies or fads, and no static about the use of adequate pain relief measures if and when you need them.

Carol Burnett described labor as similar to pulling your lower lip up over your head. Joan Rivers described it as a scream! Other mothers have described it as the joyous fulfillment of a fantastic lifetime urge. Whatever—to each her own—just remember this: You may wish to sing like Ella, dance like Ginger, write like Daphne, act like Meryl, gymnast and sell batteries like Mary Lou, run nations like Margaret, but you must recognize that there are realistic personal limitations on all these goals and those limitations must be faced. True, they need to be tested all the time. But they are still there. Learning to live comfortably against the leading edge of your personal limitations will promote a healthier, more fulfilling existence for you.

So it is with labor and delivery. Work comfortably within your own framework, comparing yourself with no one and allowing no one to compare you to anyone else or set your limitations or your goals. Thus, you will do what makes you happy and fulfilled, and that's what life is all about.

## HOSPITALS

Ninety-nine percent of all American deliveries occur in hospital settings. Obstetrical hospital services used to be very cold, isolated, sterile environments where visitors were not welcome and doctors were kings. Now, believe me, there were good, non-pompous reasons for all this. Before antibiotics, infection was one of the greatest maternal cripplers and killers. To prevent infection, labor wards were isolated from other hospital areas and strict sterile technique was used throughout. This infection threat is now largely gone, of course, but old habits are hard to break. In this case, consumer resistance helped to speed things up. Preparedness classes and modern anesthesia techniques also helped make the labor wards more tolerable for all and so gradually they have opened up and at some times resemble a church picnic.

Also changing is the fundamental decor and composition of most labor areas. Birthing rooms, decorated much like a combined bedroom and sitting room, are available in most hospitals. In such rooms, labor and delivery can take place with very little alterations. Sometimes the bed breaks to form a delivery table and in other instances it can be altered to form a type of delivery chair. This later technique is coming increasingly into vogue. In all environments you still will most likely have continuous monitoring (see pages 261–66) and an established intravenous line. After delivery the baby, if well, stays with you for bonding and nursing.

During the short postpartum stay that we are becoming accustomed to, most hospitals have arrangements for father and baby to stay with you. Although this may be more closeness than you want, it is worth a try. It is not unusual for celebration dinners with champagne to be part of this new hospital care as well, but your baby is excluded from this feast.

Many other subtle and remarkable changes are taking place in modern delivery suites, and hopefully you will get to see them all.

## THE PLACENTA

As you already know, the placenta is made up of chorionic villi, which at one time surrounded the whole embryo and from which chorionic sampling may be done in early pregnancy. As pregnancy advances, the villi recede to an area the size of a Granny Smith pie and become firmly attached to the uterine wall. This is the placenta. Through the chorionic villi, fetal blood circulates and is oxygenated and fed while carbon dioxide and other wastes are removed. The umbilical cord, of course, carries the fetal blood out and back. The placenta has about nine months to live and thus at full term shows all the degenerating tissue changes present in any other senior citizen. Although the placenta is usually inspected and discarded at delivery, it is sometimes saved and used, its substance preserved to be later extracted into certain hormones and antibodies.

The placenta has several known functions: It exchanges gases, food, and wastes; it produces many hormones, but chiefly chorionic gonadotropin, progesterone, and estrogen, and at term, it produces a prostglandin substance in sufficient amount to initiate labor. Recent evidence has suggested that the amniotic system is more involved than the placenta in this labor-initiating role.

Many abnormal placental conditions may occur. Here are but a few:

⚬ It may be located low in the uterine cavity (placenta previa) and obstruct the birth canal, causing early and dangerous bleeding.

⚬ It may age prematurely and cause fetal growth retardation and/or fetal distress.

⚬ It may separate prematurely and produce a sudden catastrophe.

⚬ It may undergo extensive degenerative changes, losing all its normal architecture, and grow at a fantastic rate, destroying the fetus as it goes. Sometimes no fetus is ever seen. This is called a hydatid mole. It can be diagnosed by ultrasound and by HCG blood levels. It is usually removed at once. Very rarely it can cause a once very deadly cancer—choriocarcinoma—now treatable with anticancer drugs.

⚬ It may grow totally adherent to the uterus (placenta accreta), even burrow through it on rare occasions. Treatment unfortunately requires a hysterectomy.

In sum, the placenta is a remarkable entity of fantastic potential.

## AMNIOTIC FLUID

Circulating within the amniotic sac, amniotic fluid gradually increases as term is approached and then begins to decrease gradually, more rapidly if postmaturity exists. The usual maximum amount is around a quart (1000–1500 cc's), but there are wide variations.

From whence does it come? Most surely it is secreted by the amniotic sac in the main. It also, of course, picks up more and more fetal urine as time goes by.

Where does it go? Most of it disappears down the fetal throat and into the stomach.

How rapidly does it circulate? The water is replaced every two or three hours, the electrolytes somewhat slower.

What does it do? The complete role of amniotic fluid is as yet unknown. Of course, it cushions the fetus and keeps it at a very constant temperature. Moreover, it allows space for fetal movements to take place. Most recently, it has been identified as the source of the prostaglandin that initiates labor. The fetus itself signals the amniotic prostaglandin secretion, which in turn signals the mother's body to initiate labor. Thus the fetus controls its own destiny!

Problems have been associated with amniotic fluid. They are:

  ○ Hydramnios. This condition exists when there are excessive amounts of amniotic fluid present, sometimes massive amounts. Generally it is associated with congenital malformations, diabetes, hypertension of pregnancy, and multiple pregnancies. It is an unwelcome sign.

  ○ Oligohydramnios. This too is an unwelcome sign. Insufficient amounts of amniotic fluid generally signal a congenital problem or a very post-term pregnancy.

The diagnosis of both these conditions is confirmed by ultrasound and an excellent example of hydramnios is seen in the section of photographs following page 118. Oligohydramnios and hydramnios are treated as part of the conditions with which they coexist.

As a matter of teleological interest, amniotic fluid closely resembles the chemical composition of seawater.

## GENETICS

Although there is a very complete review of genetics and genetic study techniques on pages 249–50, you may want to read a little bit about it here since it is a very important primelife topic.

Gregor Johann Mendel, an Austrian botanist and a Roman Catholic priest, established the laws of heredity during his experiments with garden peas over 100 years ago. His work lay unnoticed till this century, but it now has become the firm basis of all genetic study.

It is clear that all inherited human characteristics are encoded on genes which reside on the twenty-three paired chromosomes found in the nucleus of each cell in our bodies. Twenty-two pair are autosomes and one pair represent the sex chromosomes. One member of each pair comes from each partner in the union.

The union of the egg and sperm which unites the chromosome singletons into pairs seems to get stickier and stickier as we age, and thus primelife mothers have an increasing risk of abnormal chromosome unions and therefore abnormal embryos. Two modern techniques are available to detect such abnormalities— one technique is in wide use, the other strictly limited to a few chosen obstetrical units in this country.

    ° Amniocentesis is a widely available method of genetic embryo study and is usually done about the fifteenth week of pregnancy. The results—which may take several weeks to procure—are very accurate. The risks are minimal. (See pages 250–52.)

    ° Chorionic villi sampling is still restricted in the United States. It has the advantage of being accomplished in very early pregnancy with quick preliminary results. It is not, however, as safe as amniocentesis, and its accuracy is not yet as good. However, it will in time probably replace amniocentesis. (See pages 252–53.)

## SEX DETERMINATION

Here are some things everyone needs to know:

    ° The sex of a child is dependent on the fertilizing sperm's genetic structure. If it is a Y, there will be a boy; an X, a girl. Everyone knows that.

- Many more boys are conceived than girls but fail to make it. More ectopics are male. Nevertheless, there are still more boy babies than girl babies.

- The percentage of male births increases during wars and certain natural disasters such as floods, famines, and the like.

- The rich have more sons; primelife parents more girls.

- Very active sexual parents are more likely to have boys. No comment.

- Fertility drugs (e.g., clomiphene) produce more girls.

## Sex selection

For any number of reasons the preselection of a desired sex has eternally intrigued us, and indeed, much scientific work is directed in that area. In some instances, there is good medical reason for achieving these goals since certain devastating inherited disorders are linked to the sex chromosomes—hemophilia, for instance, is linked to the Y (male) chromosome.

In some laboratories, male- and female-producing sperm are separated by centrifuge since there is a difference in their weights. Other experiments rely on the ability of the male sperm to swim faster and more actively than the female and so separation is achieved by having the sperm work out in a starchy gel—like swimming in olive oil. Other labs use other techniques, and yes, gradually separation is being achieved. Some activists are opposed to this work, lamenting to all that when a choice is offered, a male will always be the first one selected and since the first baby in a family is always treated best—well, you can figure out the rest. In actual fact, things have not worked out that way with couples participating in these studies.

## Confirming fetal sex

No one spins a wedding band on a string over the abdomen anymore to predetermine an unborn child's sex, although it used to be a pretty popular party pastime. There are now several reliable tests to confirm exactly what everyone is dying to know, but such tests cannot be used just to satisfy curiosity.

○ Chorionic villi sampling. (See pages 252–53.) This as-yet-limited placental sampling procedure is virtually 100 percent correct as early as the seventh week of pregnancy.

○ Amniocentesis. (See pages 250–52.) Amniotic fluid removed from around the fetus during the fifteenth week of pregnancy or thereabouts will yield the correct sex identification a few weeks later.

○ Ultrasound. (See pages 258–61.) Modern equipment employed by a skilled ultrasonographer is now batting about 85 percent in the sex predetermination game. It has the great advantage of being a safe procedure, while the other two carry a certain definite risk with them—as well as great expense.

Ordinarily it is perhaps better not to know. Uncertainty is a prime moving force in the universe. Learn to live with it.

## TWINS

It is not likely that any primelife mother is going to have quintuplets. Even with the use of modern fertility medication, that harvest is uncommon. You read about yields of six, seven, or more infants simply because these events are so rare. This is fortunate because under such circumstances healthy survival is difficult to achieve, and the medical and financial problems such litters create are more than most parents can bear. Twins are another story.

Although, for some reason, the incidence of twins is declining worldwide, primelife mothers are slightly more likely to have twins, particularly fraternal twins. Here are some more facts about plural pregnancies:

○ The rate of twinning is supposed to be once every 80 births; of triplets, once every 6400 births ($80 \times 80$); of quads, once every 510,000 births ($80 \times 80 \times 80$); and so on up the ladder. Many things alter this formula. American blacks have a greater chance of twinning and African blacks even more so. In fact, Nigerian mothers have 40 twins in every 1000 births. Contrast this with 6.4 per thousand in the Orient.

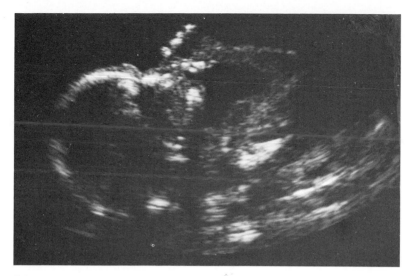

A twenty-eight-week fetus, placidly lying on its back and sucking its thumb.

An absolutely incredible picture of a fetal hand at thirty-two weeks. There is no need to identify any of the anatomy; it is very clear.

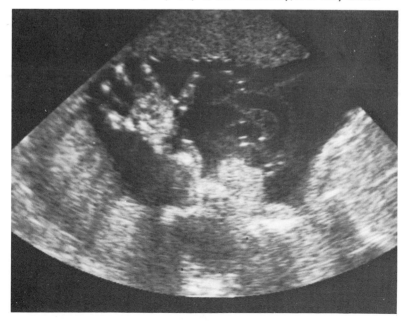

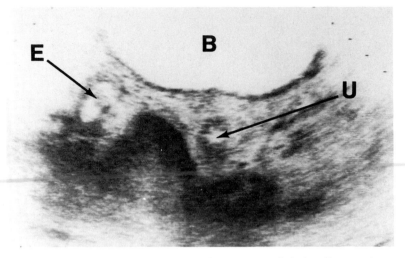

An ectopic pregnancy (E) of about seven weeks' duration and un-ruptured. The uterus (U) contains a false sac, which can be very misleading. The big white area is a full bladder (B). In this real-time scan, the fetal heart could be seen beating.

A ruptured ectopic pregnancy (E) with free blood in the abdomen (A). The large white area is a full bladder (B).

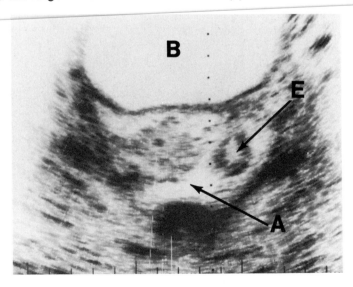

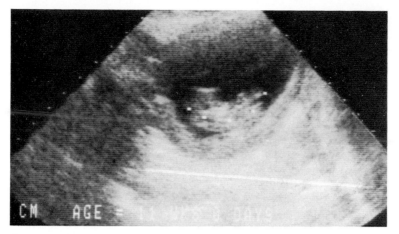

One of the most accurate ways of determining fetal age in the early months is to measure from the top of the fetal head (crown) to the rump. In this picture, the most distant dots give that measurement and the fetal age, almost to the day.

Another measurement to determine fetal age and development is the bi-parietal diameter (BPD). Here it is measured between the two stars, giving us a fetal age that is accurate to the day.

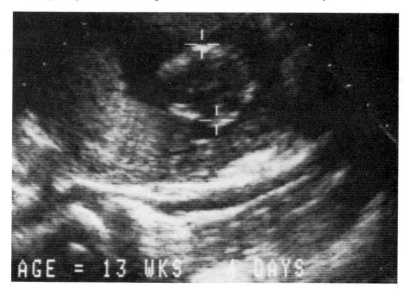

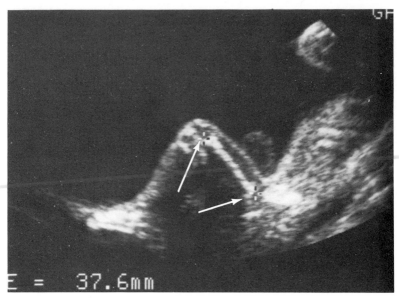

An unusually clear fetal profile. The femur is being measured between the stars and indicates a twenty-one-week fetus.

A facial profile of the same infant as in the photograph above.

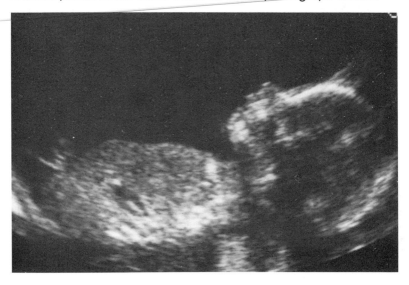

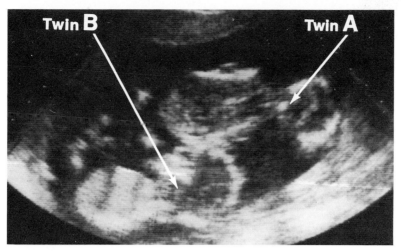

Looking like two bowling pins lying side by side are a pair of fifteen week twins.

An ultrasound recording of fetal heart beats (FB), indicating 133 beats per minute.

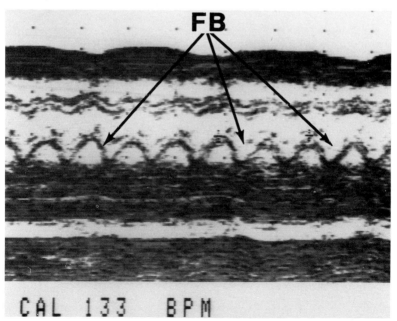

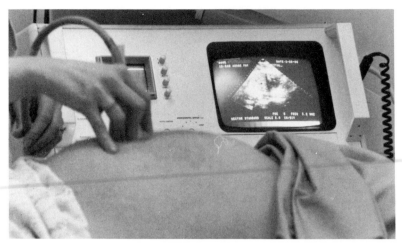

The transducer in an ultrasound examination scans the abdomen, and the picture on the screen is a transverse slice at the exact level of the scan. In this case, the screen shows the area just slightly above the level of the scan seen in the following photograph. Nine weeks later, this mother was delivered of a very healthy male child, just as the scan indicated.

A thirty-week pregnancy showing the penis (P) and the scrotum (S) containing two testicles.

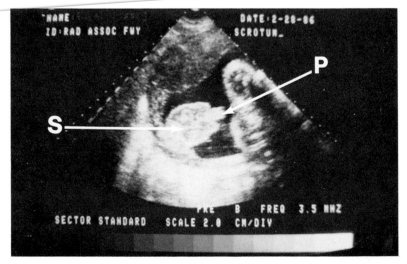

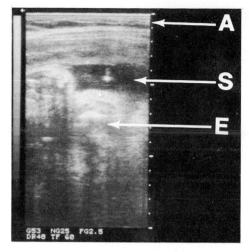

An actual amniocentesis being performed at fifteen weeks. The abdominal wall (A) is at the upper edge of the picture. The black area in the upper third is the amniotic fluid sac (S). Beneath it lies the fetus (E). The little star-shaped beam in the center of the amniotic fluid is the tip of the long needle used to aspirate away the amniotic fluid sample.

A fetus (F) at thirty-five weeks surrounded by excessive amounts of amniotic fluid (A). This is called hydramnios and is often associated with serious congenital and other fetal problems. In this case, there was obstruction in the fetal stomach that interrupted the amniotic circulation. The obstruction was thus anticipated and relieved surgically after birth.

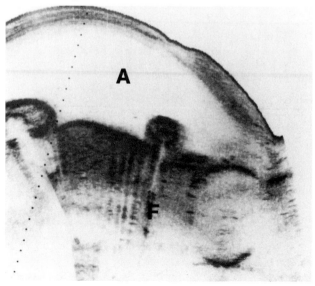

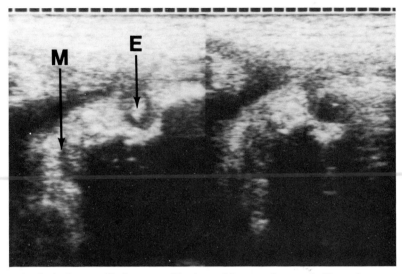

A baby's face with the eye (E) closed in one frame (left) and open in the other. The mouth (M) is clearly seen. Is it smiling?

An ultrasound shadow cast by a fetal face.

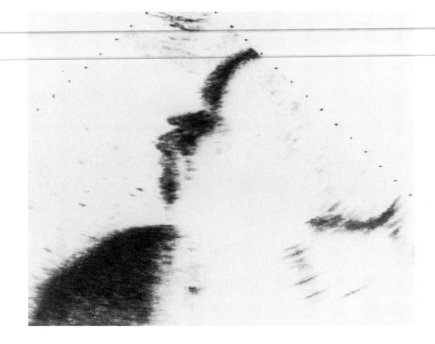

○ Identical twins come from one egg which becomes two embryos at its first cleavage. The rate of identical twinning is unaffected by any factor and continues at the same rate worldwide.

○ Fraternal twins developing from two eggs are more common in primelife mothers and in families with twin histories. Generations are not skipped. The rate of fraternal twinning varies worldwide and is decreasing.

○ Superfetation can cause fraternal twinning with different due dates. This is because fertilization and implantation may occur in a uterus that already contains a pregnancy from the previous cycle. This is a fact.

Superfecundation can produce twins from separate eggs, ovulated about the same time, but fertilized at separate sexual encounters, by the same or another male. This too is a fact.

○ Upper multiples of three, four, five, and on generally come from several eggs. Thus, the Dionnes came from three eggs with two sets of identical twins and one fraternal loner.

○ Distinguishing identical from fraternal twins may be very easy, but sometimes requires sensitive laboratory analysis—even chromosome cultures. But generally:

Twins of different sex are of course fraternal.

Twins in one common sac are identical.

Microscopic analysis of the membranes separating twins can aid in identifying their nature.

One placenta usually indicates identical twins. Still, identical twins can have separate placenta while the originally separate placentas of fraternal twins may merge together at some point.

The obstetrical problems of plural pregnancies are many:

○ Premature labor is the general rule with twins and up—the more babies, the earlier labor is likely to take place. Even born at full term, twins are likely to be small because after the twenty-eighth week they tend to gain more slowly than singletons.

○ There may be a significant weight difference between twins either because their nourishment was not equally provided by the placenta or because of superfetation. Identical twins are more likely to have the same weights.

° Hydramnios (excess amniotic fluid), anemia, abnormal presentations or positions, and maternal hypertension are all more likely in plural pregnancies.

° Plural pregnancies can be diagnosed with accuracy by ultrasound as early as six weeks unless, of course, they are identical and in one sac. By the eighth week, even identical twins can usually be identified. Ultrasound is further useful in monitoring the growth and development of each fetus as pregnancy progresses.

° Multiple pregnancies are very often delivered by cesarian section because of the risks to small bodies delivering vaginally and because of the frequency of abnormal presentations. You and your doctor will decide the best way to deliver on an individual basis. All twin births should be at a level II or III obstetrical unit, and all triplets and above should be delivered at a level III unit. (See page 240.)

° You will probably be advised to obtain extra rest during the last trimester. This rest is preferably carried out in bed lying on your left side because that position takes more pressure off your major abdominal blood vessels. Rest does not decrease your chances of premature labor, but it does increase the nourishment and health of your babies.

## THE Rh FACTOR

At about the time today's primelife mothers were themselves being born, Rh incompatibilities, when they occurred, produced a 50 percent fetal loss. Today that loss is in the vicinity of 5 to 6 percent because of techniques now at hand to prevent Rh sensitization. Here is how the Rh problem arises:

The Rh antigen (named after the Rhesus monkey where it was first identified) is a protein which coats the red blood cells of most (85 percent) humans. These folks are designated as Rh positive. The remaining 15 percent of us do not have that protein coating and are, of course, Rh negative. The Rh factor, like eye color, has no known value, but is the source of several medical and obstetrical problems.

When Rh negative individuals are exposed to the Rh antigen, they develop antibodies against it in accordance with their immune defense system's responsibilities, just as that system builds antibodies to polio when exposed to the polio vaccine antigen. The Rh antibodies are generally short-lived, while the polio antibodies may last a lifetime.

An Rh negative person can be exposed to Rh positive blood from a mismatched blood transfusion or during pregnancy. If an Rh negative mother is carrying an Rh positive child, any of the following circumstances delivers small amounts of an Rh positive baby's blood into the mother's circulation:

- Abortions—5 percent
- Ectopics—1 percent
- Amniocentesis—1 to 3 percent
- Term pregnancy—1 to 2 percent till delivery, 14 to 17 percent after delivery

The placental membrane is supposed to separate maternal and fetal blood at all times. This is not always so, and in any of the above circumstances, some fetal blood may indeed get into the maternal blood and so her immune system starts to work—provided again that the fetal blood is Rh positive and thus carries the antigen.

If mother does in fact become sensitized, she may have serious problems in future transfusions and the Rh positive fetus may be put into significant jeopardy because mother's Rh antibodies can cross the placenta to the fetal side and there begin to destroy (hemolyze or shrivel) fetal red blood cells. Such cell destruction produces more and more bilirubin (a breakdown product of blood which infants cannot handle in large amounts) and increasing anemia. In severe cases, fetal death in the uterus is not uncommon.

In 1968, Rh immune globulin first appeared on the market. Since that time Rh incompatibility problems have declined rapidly. The vaccine is very safe and very effective. It is given in varying doses to Rh negative mothers as follows:

° After any type of abortion.

° After an ectopic pregnancy.

° After amniocentesis procedures.

° At twenty-eight weeks of pregnancy if no Rh antibodies are detected by a Coombs' test. This is a maternal blood test which is used to follow the course of pregnancies with a potential for Rh disorders. The Coombs' test is used frequently throughout pregnancy to chart the course of Rh interactions.

° After delivery—preferably within three days and only if the maternal Coombs' test is not significantly elevated, in which case it can't be given. There is of course no need to give the vaccine if the baby is Rh negative. All babies of Rh negative mothers should have a blood type, Coombs' test, and certain other tests performed on their umbilical cord blood drawn at the time of delivery.

Even with this special care, Rh interactions still take place in pregnancy and jeopardizes the infant's survival. Under such circumstances, it may be necessary as pregnancy advances to do frequent amniocentesis procedures since amniotic fluid mirrors the amount of bilirubin that circulates in the infant's blood. It may also be necessary to transfuse the infant while it is still in the uterus. The above procedures are very difficult and require expert help. Therefore, they are best carried out in a level III maternity unit. (See page 240.) Fortunately, these pregnancies are now, thanks to the vaccine, very rare.

Some further information:

° Unless an Rh negative mother has been previously sensitized to the Rh factor by an abortion or ectopic pregnancy untreated by the vaccine, or has had a mismatched blood transfusion, her first full-term pregnancy is not likely to be threatened by Rh complications. She should still receive the vaccine at twenty-eight weeks and after delivery of an Rh positive child in order to protect the next pregnancy.

° The Rh vaccine given at twenty-eight weeks—or anytime—will not harm an Rh negative infant.

° Rh immune globulin is a product derived from pooled

human blood serum. There is absolutely no evidence that it can transmit AIDS or any other virus that may be found in *untreated* pooled human blood.

○ Father's blood type should be determined. If he is Rh negative, then all children will be Rh negative and there are only the problems of raising them. If, on the other hand, father is Rh positive, it may be possible for him to sire both Rh negative and Rh positive offsprings. It depends upon his genetic constitution, which can be determined if necessary.

○ Rh negative women who plan to be sterilized following delivery may not see the necessity of taking a postdelivery vaccine, which is, as stated, to protect future pregnancies. Nevertheless, she should take the vaccine for three reasons:

○ The sterilization may fail. There is no perfect technique.

○ Pregnancy may become desirable again in the future and most sterilization procedures are today reversible.

○ The vaccine eliminates antibodies that could be a potential transfusion hazard should one be necessary in some disorder.

ABO blood incompatibility is a rare, generally mild blood reaction, which involves the major blood groups only.

○ It is mild and fetal loss rarely occurs.

○ Mothers whose blood type is O, A, or B may be involved.

○ Unlike the Rh interaction, 50 percent take place in the first pregnancy.

○ There are no predictive tests such as the Coombs' test in following blood interaction.

○ The amount of bilirubin that accumulates is much less and can usually be managed after birth by special light treatments in the nursery.

○ A warning here: If you take your baby home early as most families are doing nowadays, be sure and report to your pediatrician any evidence of jaundice or yellowing of your baby's skin. This represents excess bilirubin, which again must be light treated.

# TORCH COMPLEX

This term is used in obstetrics to describe a mixed set of infections that have but one thing in common—they are known to be damaging to babies before, during, or soon after birth. The term is derived as follows:

**T** — Toxoplasmosis

**O** — Others: hepatitis B, Beta streptococcus, influenza, mumps, varicella (chicken pox), and other infectious disorders, such as chlamydia, as yet unclassified

**R** — Rubella (German measles)

**C** — Cytomegalovirus (CMV)

**H** — Herpes virus II

Many of these infectious diseases are discussed in other areas of the book, but are brought together here for a number of reasons:

○ Clinically, the effect that these agents have upon newborns is indistinguishable. Only special laboratory tests can tell them apart.

○ Taken together, they have a significant impact on newborn well-being.

○ The symptoms may not appear at once and can have long-term damaging effects.

○ Many times the maternal infection is very mild, even unnoticed or passed off as a virus or a bad cold and then forgotten, and becomes hard to trace.

All this sounds very frightening, but while as many as 15 percent of all pregnancies may be involved with a member of the TORCH family, only 12 percent of these may sustain fetal structural damage as a result of their involvement. If the infection occurs in the first trimester, generally the TORCH involvement might affect the eyes, heart, neurological system, or the blood-forming system of the fetus. In the later months generally the problems are more subtle—small-for-dates babies, slow to develop, mental retardation, and so forth.

Here follows a brief description of the TORCH diseases that

are not covered elsewhere in this book. More comprehensive and extensive data is available from your doctor, to whom you should report any unusual infectious illnesses while you are pregnant.

## Toxoplasmosis

This disease, which produces a flulike illness in humans, is contracted in one of two ways:

○ Cats. About 1 percent of the outside cat population is infected with toxoplasmosis at any given time. They shed the organism in their stools for a few weeks and then are free of the disease—at least for a while. They get it from eating infected rodents or from other cats' stools so:

If you have an inside cat, it is probably free of the disease. Don't change its litter box, though.

If you have an inside/outside cat, don't pet it or change its litter box.

If you have an outside cat, leave it alone.

If you get a flulike infection, send your cat to the vet for a toxoplasmosis titer and ask your doctor to do one on you. Many obstetricians do such titers routinely at the first visit so you would then be provided with a baseline level to use as a comparative source.

Keep all cats out of your kitchen.

○ Infected pork or lamb. This is definitely the source of most toxoplasmosis in other countries and may be so in our own. These meats should be either well cooked before consumption or should be frozen solid for at least four hours before they are thawed and cooked.

It might be wise for women who work in veterinary clinics or in processing meat at any level to have a regular toxoplasmosis test drawn while they are pregnant.

There are medications that can be given for toxoplasmosis after the first trimester. They certainly reduce the risk of congenital symptoms in the newborn. Toxoplasmosis can be transmitted very rarely by blood transfusions, but you would not have a blood transfusion unless your life was on the line from some much more drastic complication than toxoplasmosis.

## Hepatitis B

This common virus is discussed under immunization (see page 80). It is rapidly yielding to preventive measures.

## Beta hemolytic streptoccocus

This bacteria, which is incriminated in a number of obstetrical problems, is covered on page 99.

## Influenza and mumps

Growing evidence incriminates a number of virus disorders in long-term fetal and newborn problems. In certain cases this relationship is clear—rubella, for instance—as you will read below. In others, only a thread of evidence holds the story together, but it appears that once viruses invade our bodies, many of them take up residence there forever, altering the host area in ways that may not become apparent for years.

As an example, chicken pox, supposed to come and go in a short visit during childhood, may some forty or more years later break forth in an exceedingly painful march across any peripheral nerve of its choice, leaving behind a track of exquisitely tender red spots called shingles. You've heard of that. Even live attenuated virus that halts deadly diseases (live polio vaccine, for instance) may return in later years to haunt some host in some temporary ways. This is not to say that the vaccines should not be given—they should.

So it is that some forms of influenza and mumps may, if acquired during pregnancy, have some later effect on the infants so exposed. Mumps vaccine should be given early in life and influenza vaccine—reformulated every few years—should be administered to pregnant women in an epidemic situation.

## Chicken pox

This is probably the most contagious of all diseases and is usually very mild, even though it is a distant cousin of herpes II. Most people are immune to chicken pox but about one mother in 7,500 contracts it during pregnancy. There is no treatment, but the baby must be watched for certain long-term effects.

## Rubella—German measles

There is no doubt that the time has come for this disease. It can be—and should be—eliminated from the face of the earth as smallpox was. The vaccine is available and safe, and every child should be vaccinated and, if necessary, revaccinated later in life. But epidemics keep cropping up around the country, the last one in 1964 costing us billions of dollars and damaging untold infants in the uterus. Rubella contracted by the mother in the first trimester can maim her child for life, so badly and so commonly that abortion is sometimes recommended for mothers so infected. Further:

○ Vaccinate your children. This is stated to be a safe approach even while you are pregnant.

○ Do not get vaccinated while pregnant. If you accidentally do, consult your doctor about it.

○ If you have never been vaccinated or your immunity is low (check with your doctor), then you should be vaccinated before you leave the hospital after delivery. This should be done even if you nurse, although there has been recent criticism of this technique. Your doctor will know the latest on this subject.

○ Practice strict birth control for at least sixty days after vaccination. That's why when you're in the hospital is a good time to get vaccinated.

German measles is a declining viral problem but it still has the potential to ravage your pregnancy. Be on your guard about vaccination, exposure, and informing your doctor if you develop runny eyes, sore throat, swollen neck glands, and a rash.

## Cytomegalovirus

This is a fairly common sexually transmitted virus that at one time—early in the game—was thought to cause AIDS. But it doesn't. In women it generally resides in the cervix and causes few symptoms except a discharge. It can unfortunately cross the placenta during pregnancy and thus damage the infant in the TORCH tradition. Fortunately, it is rare.

There are tests available now which can demonstrate the disease's presence in mother or child, but treatment is very ineffective and a vaccine may be the final answer.

## Herpes virus II

This virus disorder is covered on pages 99–101. The new systemic treatment of herpes infections is not advisable during pregnancy.

So this is the sad litany of the TORCH complex and it unfortunately is a growing litany. It certainly is not a hopeless situation, and as you read you can see that there is a great deal that you can do to protect your baby from exposure to this terrible tribe. You can also take comfort in the fact that rarely does the offending invader get to the baby and the 1 to 2 percent attack figure—even in the exposed group—is quite accurate and comfortable.

## THE LOW BIRTH WEIGHT INFANT/PREMATURITY AND INTRAUTERINE GROWTH RETARDATION

In March 1985, a most unusual hearing by the House Subcommittee on Health and Environment was held in an auditorium at the Children's National Medical Center in Washington, D.C. The star witness—who didn't say a word—was Baby Jane Doe, a subject of great national press coverage and interest. Her physician explained that Baby Jane, born three months premature and weighing 3.5 pounds, would cost $60,000 in medical care before her release from the hospital. It was eloquent testimony to a major obstetrical and social problem of our country, the low birth weight (LBW) infant. Consider:

○ There are 250,000 LBW infants born in the United States each year.

○ The cost of their initial hospital care is often over $100,000. The total annual intensive care bill for them is $1.5 billion.

○ The duration of hospital stay of healthy term newborns averages 3.5 days. It averages 24 days for infants between 3.3 and 4.4 pounds, while infants 2.2 to 3.3 pounds at birth average 89 hospital days.

○ LBW infants who survive and enter the real world are subject to immense medical problems that make it difficult for them to cope and survive. The continued cost to society is immense.

○ Every dollar spent on prenatal care will save $3.8 down the road. Adequate prenatal care could prevent one third of all LBW deliveries.

All of the factors known to influence the LBW occurrence are listed below and not in order of importance. That order will be developed as we move along. First, though, most LBW infants are generally the end result of premature labor or intrauterine growth retardation (IUGR) or both. Let's see what they are.*

## PRINCIPAL RISK FACTORS FOR LOW BIRTH WEIGHT

○ Demographic Risks
  – Age (less than 17; over 34)
  – Race (black)
  – Low socioeconomic status
  – Unmarried
  – Low level of education

○ Medical Risks Predating Pregnancy
  – Parity (0 or more than 4)
  – Low weight for height
  – Genitourinary anomalies/surgery
  – Selected diseases such as diabetes, chronic hypertension
  – Nonimmune status for selected infections such as rubella
  – Poor obstetric history including previous low birth weight infant, multiple spontaneous abortions
  – Maternal genetic factors (such as low maternal weight at own birth)

○ Medical Risks in Current Pregnancy
  – Multiple pregnancy
  – Poor weight gain

*Source: American College of Obstetricians and Gynecologists, "IOM Publishes Conclusions on Low Birth Weight," *ACOG Newsletter* 29(4):5, 1985.

- Short interpregnancy interval
- Hypotension
- Hypertension/preeclampsia/toxemia
- Selected infections such as symptomatic bacteriuria, rubella, and cytomegalovirus
- First or second trimester bleeding
- Placental problems such as placenta previa, abruptio placentae
- Hyperemesis
- Oligohydramnios/polyhydramnios
- Anemia/abnormal hemoglobin
- Isoimmunization
- Fetal anomalies
- Incompetent cervix
- Spontaneous premature rupture of membranes
° Behavioral and Environmental Risks
- Smoking
- Poor nutritional status
- Alcohol and other substance abuse
- DES exposure and other toxic exposures, including occupational hazards
- High altitude
° Health Care Risks
- Absent or inadequate prenatal care
- Latrogenic prematurity
° Evolving Concepts of Risk
- Stress, physical and psychological
- Uterine irritability
- Events triggering uterine contractions
- Cervical changes detected before onset of labor
- Selected infections such as mycoplasmosis and chlamydia
- Inadequate plasma volume expansion
- Progesterone deficiency

# PREMATURE LABOR

Regardless of the cause, premature labor is that which occurs before the thirty-seventh week of pregnancy or which produces a child weighing less than 2500 grams (5 pounds, 8 ounces). Since one out of every ten pregnancies end in premature labor, it is clearly an important obstetrical and national health problem. The causes are found in the list just noted. But please note these are not listed in order of importance or frequency. Before we do that we need to eliminate two sources of prematurity that muddy up the water a bit.

- Ethnic and race variations. Our society is a meld of multiple groups some of which, by their genetic constitution, have smaller babies. Many healthy full-term babies born to such groups may, by their weight alone, be designated as premature and thus affect statistical reporting.

- Obstetricians at times contribute to prematurity by delivering babies early because of circumstances that make pregnancy continuation unwise, for example, in severe hypertension of pregnancy. Premature babies thus delivered fare better outside the uterus than within, but they are still premature.

Those two factors being disposed of, we can now address the *major* causes of prematurity.

- Malnutrition.
- Absence of prenatal care.
- Adolescent and primelife mothers.
- Alcohol, tobacco, and drugs.
- Maternal diseases (diabetes, hypertension, etc.).
- Uterine malformations due to tumors, congenital defects, or to an incompetent cervical canal.
- Abnormal placental location or early placental separation.

Now, a special word about primelife mothers and prematurity. The statistics which say you are a leading candidate for premature problems do not reflect the whole story. Many of the figures are gathered from clinics seeing older pregnant women who are chronically undernourished, habituated to one thing or another, and who have had little or no prenatal care. Unless your primelife pregnancy is already complicated by a medical problem such as diabetes or hypertension, or by a disorder of uterine structure, you should expect no problems from prematurity provided you eat properly, have adequate prenatal care, avoid tobacco, alcohol, drugs, and toxic environments, and comply reasonably with reasonable instructions.

## Arresting labor

When, in your management, premature labor appears to be a possibility, you should receive particular instructions for self-care to help prevent its onset. Also, you should be aware of the very early signs that could indicate the onset of premature labor. (These are lower abdominal cramping, backache, increased pelvic pressure, and blood or mucous in the vaginal secretions.) However, once premature labor begins, every effort is made to stop it, provided that the membranes have not ruptured (see pages 134–135) and that the uterine environment is not hostile to the infant. There are two agents generally used in attempting to arrest labor:

○ Ritodrine, a powerful beta-adrenergic agent, which has now been approved for use in the prevention of premature labor. It must be used in a hospital setting where both mother and baby can be monitored very adequately. Close observation of the maternal cardiovascular system is a must. Treatment with ritodrine is initially by the intravenous route and, if successful, continued treatment can be given as oral tablets and patients can even be discharged home to continue oral treatment.

○ Magnesium sulfate is epsom salts, which was once used as a powerful laxative—and it was! Given intravenously, magnesium sulfate will many times arrest labor. If it becomes effective, it is not, for obvious reasons, easy to take orally. But it can be done. Magnesium sulfate is also a very powerful drug and close maternal-fetal monitoring is essential when it is first introduced.

These agents are reasonably effective in arresting premature labor when there are no complicating factors, and they have reduced fetal mortality and morbidity in a remarkable way. Even when premature labor can only be temporarily arrested, these drugs are of value by providing us with a few days lag time and can arrest labor long enough for us to speed up fetal lung maturity. This can often be accomplished with the use of cortisone administered to the mother over a forty-eight-hour period.

## Intrauterine growth retardation

IUGR represents another major portion of the LBW calamity. Growth-retarded babies are small for their gestational age and are the result of an intrauterine accident of some sort. Depending upon the type of accident, there are two types of IUGR.

o Symmetrical. The whole body is equally reduced in size. This growth retardation is generally due to a genetic factor or to an intrauterine insult or injury sustained in early pregnancy—for instance, TORCH (see pages 124–28) infections, toxins (Love Canal, for example), and high altitude environments. After birth, these infants are generally slow to grow and develop, and are more likely to have neurological problems.

o Asymmetrical. In this state, the body is usually reduced in size more than the head. IUGR here is generally a placental disorder preventing adequate fetal nourishment. It is found in association with maternal diseases (hypertension, etc.), tobacco, alcohol, and drugs.

Thus, because of IUGR many infants are born weighing less than 2500 grams but are not premature by dates. Further, it is equally true that some babies with a birth weight greater than 2500 grams may also be growth retarded but not by definition premature.

IUGR is diagnosed almost exclusively by ultrasound studies. Obstetricians maintain a high index of suspicion when uterine enlargement fails to keep pace with the normal parameters expected as pregnancy advances. Particularly watched are mothers who are at greater risk for IUGR. But the final diagnosis is made by ultrasound (see pages 258–61). This technique is also used to follow the course of IUGR and to assist in determining the timing and the method of delivery.

## Premature rupture of the membranes (PROM)

The amniotic sac looks like a balloon filled with water—except it is filled with an infant. When that sac ruptures spontaneously before full term, it causes one third of all premature deliveries and sets a hazardous chain of events in motion.

° The fetus is now connected with the world, and infections of various sorts can and do get into its space and body. Generally, the longer the time lapse between rupture and delivery, the greater the risk of infection.

° The umbilical cord may come down (prolapse) and present an immediate risk of fetal death from strangulation if the cord becomes pinched. Generally this accident is associated with an abnormal fetal presentation—not an unusual companion of PROM. Fortunately, cord prolapse is not a common event.

° Labor generally follows and most infants have been delivered within seventy-two hours of the event, often drastically premature.

Why does this serious event occur? Currently, it is held that certain bacteria which can colonize in the vagina are the culprits which erode away the membrane walls and cause them to rupture. A Beta hemolytic streptococcus is the main suspect at this time but there are others. No matter what the cause, the rate of occurrence remains unchanged over the years.

What to do?

° Fetal assessment. Ultrasound studies are obtained to determine fetal age with accuracy, and amniocentesis is often performed to help assess fetal lung maturity and also the possibility of intra-amniotic infection.

° Maternal observation. This helps determine the possibility of intra-amniotic and therefore intrauterine infection since mother shares that infectious risk with her babe. External abdominal monitoring (see pages 261–70) may further help to demonstrate the presence of fetal infection (by the fetal heart rate) and to indicate if labor has begun (by displaying uterine contractions).

Based on the data these studies yield, your doctor, in consultation with you, will decide whether it is better to empty the uterus at once or to buy a little time to try and increase fetal lung maturity with cortisone before attempting a delivery. Each case must be decided on its own individual characteristics and it would be a mistake to try and give you hard and fast guidelines. Your doctor will know how to advise you should you have to face this challenging pregnancy complication.

## POSTMATURITY

Prolongation of pregnancy beyond forty-two weeks involves between 5 to 10 percent of all pregnancies, but not all of them are to worry about. They are all a drag to the owner, that's for sure. Friends, relatives, and even the mailman will bug you daily and your baby will do it night and day. Here are some things to dwell upon while you wait:

o Postmaturity should be clearly documented. The last menstrual period is often (25 percent of the time) *not* an accurate indicator. Early ultrasound and very early pregnancy testing offer much more reliable data in setting the exact due date. It is becoming clear that all primelife mothers should have an early ultrasound procedure for this and other purposes. Recorded observations of fetal growth, development, and movement throughout pregnancy are other ways of evaluating true postmaturity.

o Many pregnancies should probably not be continued beyond forty-two weeks. These include breeches, proven fetal inactivity, abnormal stress or nonstress tests, very large babies, hypertension, diabetes or pregnancy diabetes, decreased amniotic fluid volume, or excessive placental aging. Many times interruption of these pregnancies is advised well before forty-two weeks.

o Excluding the above conditions, postmaturity is of itself not always harmful to mother or baby. What must be watched for constantly are signs of placental senescence or aging.

There comes a point—and it often comes *sooner* in primelife pregnancies—where placental transfer is no longer sufficient to nourish the fetus. That is when labor should be induced or a cesarian section performed. The method of delivery depends upon a number of factors including cervical ripeness, fetal position, maternal health, and other factors. You and your obstetrician will settle all this between you.

° A child delivered truly postmature—be it small or large—is generally lean with little subcutaneous fat. It is also likely to have more hair and more facial expression. Such babies are generally not as healthy to begin with, and often have sleep disturbances.

° Postmaturity used to be treated expectantly—"when an apple is ripe, it will fall" was the doctrine. You don't need to be a fruit grower to know that's not always so. Anyway, the old approach allowed some pretty long pregnancies to take place. The longest documented—well, almost documented—pregnancy? Three hundred twenty-five days! Think about that for a while, particularly if you are waiting.

## CESARIAN SECTION

Whole books could be and have been written about the incredible history of the cesarian operation. Every advanced culture since the beginning of recorded history has known and used the operation. Almost always it was an agonal procedure—that is, performed at the moment of maternal death in an attempt to extract a living baby since performing the operation on a living mother usually ended in her death. Well, consider it has only been in the last 200 years that any attempt was made to sew up the uterus or abdomen after the initial opening was made! And that advance was the brainchild of an American frontier surgeon.

Incidentally, Julius Caesar may have been delivered by section, but even if he was, the operation was not named after him nor he after the operation. The name of the operation is derived, however, from Roman culture, since citizens born by abdominal incisions were known as *caesons* and later as *caesares.*

At the beginning of this century, the operation still put mothers in mortal jeopardy. The operation was utilized, after all, when everything else, including days and days of labor, all manner of external and internal manipulations, bleeding, and purges, had failed. There was no blood, no sterile technique, and no antibiotics and little pain relief. The mortality rate stood at 50 percent, and that spoke highly of maternal stamina and forbearance.

Just before this midcentury, antibiotics became generally available, and combined with the use of blood, modern surgical techniques, and better obstetrical knowledge, the section mortality rate fell below 10 percent. Since that time, it has declined steadily so that there are many hospitals (and many obstetricians, including this one) that have never witnessed a death from cesarian sections—never.

Primelife mothers have the highest section rate among all mothers, so this is important reading for us. Here are the major present-day indications for the operation:

Repeat cesarian section—35 percent

Disproportion between baby and mother—28 percent

Breech (fanny) presentation—11 percent

Fetal distress—7 percent

Others—19 percent

Others includes premature rupture of membranes, prolonged pregnancy, premature labor, multiple births, hypertension, diabetes, active herpes disease, and other maternal illnesses, placenta previa, and placental separation.

The reason that more primelife mothers are sections is that they are more likely to have problems of fetal distress and the Others listed above.

Hospitals and doctors used to be judged by their section rate—the lower, the better. They still are so judged, but to a lesser extent. So the judgment process is partly based on a throwback to the dangerous days of the operation and to fixed thinking in the "old ways" context.

In recent years, the incidence of C-section has been climbing steadily and has been a cause of private and public concern. Thus the section rate of a "good hospital" in 1970 was around 7 percent. Today that same hospital probably has a 20 to 25 percent section rate. (Primelife mothers usually run about 5 percentage points above the average so they would now have a 25 to 30 percent rate.)

Why the concern? Well, the questions are twofold. First, are we making obstetrical cripples of all these mothers by sectioning them? Second, why is it suddenly necessary to section with increasing frequency an increasingly healthy population of women?

Both questions can be answered with the same data as you already know. We used to avoid sections whenever possible because of the long history of associated morbidity and mortality as recorded above. It was hard to change our antisection conditioned responses and it had been taught for generations that any way to get the baby out through the vagina was a better way. Thus, there were any number of difficult forceps deliveries, breech deliveries, and multiple birth deliveries, all to prevent a section. Moreover, no one would consider a cesarian operation for a tiny premature baby that could literally fall out of the vagina even though the trip could still be damaging to its weakly protected brain. Fetal concerns, then, definitely had to take a backseat to maternal welfare. And at that time it was a correct judgment.

But now cesarian sections are relatively safe for mothers and infinitely better for the infants in the distressful situations we have just described. Quoting directly from a 1986 report by the National Institute of Neurological and Communicative Disorders and Stroke, "increased use of Cesarian section and decreased use of the obstetric forceps have substantially reduced birth trauma as a cause of cerebral palsy, mental retardation and epilepsy amongst infants and children."

So the following now might be the statistics of a local well-regulated hospital.

|  | 1970 | 1985 |
| --- | --- | --- |
| C-Sections | 7% | 22% |
| Operative deliveries | 20% | 2% |
| Total | 27% | 24% |

Thus, the total percentage of operative deliveries has remained static but cesarian deliveries to insure fetal well-being as far as possible have increased, while difficult and dangerous vaginal operations have decreased.

The other part of the question—are we making obstetrical cripples out of these mothers?—is a valid concern. Are we by increasing the section rate condemning more and more mothers to repeat cesarian section with its consequent risks and are we limiting their family size at the same time? Let's see.

"Once a section, always a section" is a dictum, like so many others concerning sections, that no longer applies. A repeat cesarian procedure can be avoided if:

> o The condition requiring the first section no longer exists in a subsequent pregnancy—for example, placenta previa (placenta beneath child in the uterus), which is a one-time accident of nature.

> o A low transverse incision into the uterus was used for the first section and it healed well without infection.

> o The coming trial of labor is conducted in a tertiary care center (see pages 240–41) where equipment, anesthesia, operating rooms, and support systems are instantly available twenty-four hours each day.

> o If you have given informed consent.

Under such circumstances, from 50 to 80 percent success is achieved in various centers, without increase in the fetal or maternal morbidity. The failures, of course, do not indicate that something happened to mother or baby. It simply means that the trial of labor failed for whatever reason and repeat section was resorted to.

The risk of a cesarian section has been somewhat overdone. In a private, competent setting, maternal mortality associated with cesarian section has reached the vanishing point. Under the same circumstances morbidity (fever and other postoperative complications) have equally been reduced to fractional percentage points. In thirty-five years of practice, none of my patients died from a cesarian section—as a matter of fact, no patients delivered by cesarian section in my two hospitals by any of our obstetricians ever died in that thirty-five years. I have never seen such a death—ever. Now, then, university teaching hospitals may have less reassuring statistics but you must remember they usually have a larger group of disadvantaged mothers who, for many reasons, some theirs, some society's, are subject to the most severe complications of pregnancy that often challenge the wits and wisdom of the great obstetrical masters responsible for their care at these teaching centers. You, however, are both taking and getting good care and the former is the more important one.

Finally, do sections limit your family size? Most often they do not. Your income and your coping ability play a much larger role and besides, a primelife mother doesn't have a long enough reproductive life span to have a large family anyway! Sometimes associated medical risk factors—diabetes or hypertension, for instance—will limit your family size, but modern surgical and intraoperative care is such that there is usually no reason to limit the number of repeat sections because of obstetrical risk factors. Coping risks are something else again! Remember, they are all going to be teenagers someday.

I have had the privilege of repeating the cesarian operation six times for one patient without any problems, but there are other obstetricians who have successfully repeated the procedure even more often.

What is the operation like? If you and your obstetrician have decided that a planned section before labor is in your best interests, then you come to the hospital as for any other surgical procedure. You arrive the night before or the morning of surgery, have your abdomen clipped or perhaps shaved, have some blood work done, and proceed to a holding area of some sort where an intravenous line is established. If, on the other hand, you have been in the hospital laboring or waiting when the decision is reached, you may have already had some of these things done. And if you are in labor, you may already have an epidural anesthetic started as well.

There are two major anesthetics in general use for the cesarian operation:

° Conduction (epidural or spinal) anesthesia. These "block" anesthetics are probably the most common in use today. Administered into the back, they produce temporary numbness and paralysis in the lower extremities. They and all obstetrical anesthetics are discussed in more detail farther on (see pages 161–67).

○ General anesthesia. These, whether given intravenously or by inhalation, produce deep sleep. They too are discussed in the next chapter.

Once satisfactory anesthesia has been obtained, a retention catheter is placed in the bladder, and the abdomen is washed with antiseptic solutions and covered with surgical drapes—except for the operative site! The surgery begins:

○ Either a vertical or transverse incision may be used. The transverse takes a little longer to accomplish, but is cosmetically nicer and heals very well. The vertical incision, usually ending just below the navel, has the advantage of being quicker, which can sometimes be important.

○ After opening the skin and underlying fat, three distinct muscle layers must now be separated to reach the peritoneum, a thin cellophanelike membrane that envelops all abdominal contents. Once the peritoneum is opened, the uterus is at hand. Before it can be opened, however, a further layer of attached peritoneum must be stripped away from it. Now the uterus is opened from one side to the other and the baby extracted. Once it is delivered, the umbilical cord is cut and the baby is a separate entity and it is removed to a warm observation area. One of the attendants generally puts a tube into its stomach very gently and can thus aspirate any amniotic fluid that may have accumulated there before delivery.

○ At this point, the placenta is removed and inspected, the inside of the uterus inspected, and closure begins. Every layer described above is sewn back together separately, from the uterus to the skin.

○ If a tubal ligation is to be done during the surgery, it takes place after the uterus and its layer of peritoneum is sewn back in place. A ligation procedure takes very little time and does not effect the recovery time at all.

○ When the skin has been closed, a dry dressing is put in place and it's off the table and away to recovery. If all has gone well, you may have your baby with you to bond and begin breastfeeding.

There are many variations in this operation which may not fit in completely with the above description, but by and large that is what happens. A great many important details have been skipped because they are technical.

A classical cesarian section is seldom done anymore—except in a dire emergency when great speed is necessary or when the placenta is situated in the lower uterine area making the regular incision difficult. The classical scar, then, is in the upper uterus and does not heal as well as the low transverse incision. Thus, all future deliveries must, in this situation, be by repeat section.

## NURSING: ONLY THE BREAST IS GOOD ENOUGH?

Breast feeding, a mutually rewarding, healthy, and natural goal for mother and child, is making a rewarding comeback. Earlier generations forsook the intimate and innate beauty of nursing for the convenience and supposed equality of formula feeding. Even very recently a medical student being quizzed by his pediatric professor had to stretch his ingenuity to the limits to come up with five good reasons for breast over bottle. They were:

- Mother's milk is always the right temperature.
- It always contains the right amount of protein, carbohydrate, and fat.
- It is free of bacterial contamination.
- It comes in a more attractive container.
- The cats can't get to it.

Disregarding his reasoning—which didn't get him very high marks—here are the pros and cons for breast feeding:

- The first three points above are generally true. I suppose they are all true.
- There are lymphocytes, antibodies, and as yet undifferentiated proteins in mother's milk which can protect her infant against a host of communicable and infectious complications. SIDS and necrotizing enterocolitis are less likely to occur because of these protective protein factors.

○ Breast fed babies are less likely to suffer from epidemic intestinal diseases that have such high mortality rates. A substance in human milk called lactoferrin appears to protect infants from these pathological intestinal bacteria.

○ Fewer allergies, less ear disease, less obesity seem to be the rule with breasted babies.

○ The psychological benefits to both willing participants are undeniable.

○ Cow's milk has components not ideally suited for human babies. It also may be contaminated with bacteria, and, alas, with a growing number of toxic chemicals introduced into the human food chain. As an example, the very day this is being written, cow's milk is being withdrawn from grocery stores all over Arkansas because of its contamination with heptachlor. This chemical, now banned, has been used in the past to reduce insect destruction of corn. The corn involved here was to have been used to make gasahol, but somehow found its way into feeding dairy herds. Thus it is endangering us rather than our cars.

Against breast feeding:

○ Expanded career goals may make nursing a bilateral luxury that cannot be afforded. More corporations are adopting liberal maternity leave, but the corporation itself may be the lesser antagonist of your goals. That is something you have to deal with.

○ A difficult, arduous, and energy-sapping pregnancy may also make nursing a luxury you cannot afford. This is especially true if you have a continuing medical problem (diabetes, for instance) that of itself requires too much of your reserves.

○ Certain other disorders and problems preclude nursing. Even with modern vaccines, mothers who carry hepatitis B or who have active toxoplasmosis should not nurse. Also restricted are mothers on many medications, all recreational drugs, alcohol, and tobacco.

More about breasts and nursing:

° Routine mammography (breast x-rays) should be avoided in pregnancy for a number of reasons. This does not exclude, however, indicated mammography when breast disease is suspected. Breast cancer does occur during pregnancy and should be treated largely the same way as it would be at any other time. Therapeutic abortion does not improve treatment results but often early delivery is indicated if radiation or chemotherapy is contemplated. Nursing must be avoided. Primelife women who have arrested breast cancer for at least three years may consider conceiving with the advice and consent of their oncologist and obstetrician. All planned primelife pregnancies should be preceded by a screening mammogram. (See page 13.)

° The absence or relative absence of colostrum during pregnancy does not indicate that there will be a nursing problem.

° Although the breasts become engorged and edematous within forty-eight hours after delivery, the engorger is not milk. Milk makes its appearance shortly thereafter, but your baby should be put to breast as soon after delivery as possible and regularly thereafter in order to reinforce its suckling response, to bond, and to keep the pituitary-breast stimulation cycle as active as possible until the milk is in.

° Breast infections—even abscesses—can complicate nursing. Usually such infections are corrected by antibiotics and nursing can continue. Nursing shields may help spare tender nipples.

° In the event that you do not wish to nurse or for some reason cannot nurse, a variety of agents are available to help decrease the tender swollen engorged glands pulling on your chest wall. Sometimes short-duration hormones are used, but the most common medication today reduces the level of pituitary stimulation to the breasts and it takes about two weeks of treatment to terminate the cycle.

A final note on nursing: No amount of peer or grandpeer pressure should be the stimulus that leads you to nursing. No sense of obligation or duty should lead you there either. No guilt or shame should devolve upon you should you for whatever reason decide not to nurse or that you cannot nurse. Too much of a hassle has been put upon you already by any number of sources about your obligations to preparing, parenting, bonding, nursing, and giving. Don't let it all get to you. Should you be able to and want to nurse, it will be a mutually rewarding experience. Should you not, there will be no lasting benefits to anyone. Your baby can sense rejection very early.

The intensely personal subject of nursing is a difficult one for men to comment upon, no matter how compassionate and understanding they feel they may be. I leave this very sensitive area in your hands.

ooooooooooooo **THINGS TO THINK ABOUT** ooooooooooooo

Delayed triplet birth. Recent medical literature recounts a very unusual triplet pregnancy—in fact, the only one of its kind ever reported. The first triplet was born at twenty-three weeks and survived but a few hours. The second and third triplets did not follow the first and indeed they did not deliver for almost 100 more days—within two weeks of full term!

ooooooo

Rh immune globulin is a very important agent in managing Rh problem pregnancy. It is made from pooled human plasma. At this writing, it is declared to be free of any risk of AIDS contamination. Donors are thoroughly screened and the manufacturing process destroys bacteria and viruses.

ooooooo

Some interesting things about the low birth weight problem:

o Both sexual intercourse and orgasm have been singled out as a cause for premature labor—even when there is no history of previous premature labor. Sexual activity, however, is hard to classify and document. For instance, one study reveals that the average duration of coitus is thirty to forty-five minutes while another study in the same locality but in a different socioeconomic group reports an average coital duration of five minutes. Variables like that are hard to equate when studying anything.

∘ An Omaha program called Ladies in Wading encourages women to swim—or at least pool exercise—while pregnant. The theory holds that exercising in shoulder-deep water tends to promote fetal circulation and help prevent premature labor.

∘ Women resident physicians training in obstetrics tend to be at greater risk for low birth weight babies.

∘ Extramarital affairs may cause premature labor not from anxiety, but from venereal bacteria that may be brought home, transmitted, and initiate labor.

∘ A promising test for the diagnosis of true premature labor lies in the fact that fetal breathing is reduced during actual labor. Real-time ultrasound can measure breathing activity very accurately. More will develop in this area within the next few years.

Low birth weight is truly a very major public health problem. From the moment of birth such infants are disadvantaged to the extent that many of them will remain public charges as long as they live. The cost of their maintenance after birth and continuing on is an incredible financial drain upon all our resources. Much of this you already know. What to do?

∘ Adequate prenatal care, including a proper nutrition intake.

∘ Sex education in early school years and birth control assistance to halt the tide of little children having little children.

∘ Maternal compliance with what is known to cause prematurity. Tobacco, alcohol, and drug abuse rank very high as causes of LBW infants.

∘ Recognition by the obstetrician of anatomical problems that can produce repeated premature labor.

∘∘∘∘∘∘∘∘

Explaining the cesarian section rate: On all sides, obstetricians are being assailed because of the rapid increase in section rates. Fear of lawsuits, fear of bad results, bigger fees, misinterpretation of monitor signals—all and more have been leveled at us as causes of the sudden and continuing rise in section rates. Let me be candid with you. There may be some truth in all these changes but, as you have already learned, the major reason is that a cesarian section is now replacing vaginal operations as the method of handling obstructed and dangerous labors. As one goes down the other goes up and so does fetal survival and health and maternal vaginal health as well. If we went back to the old ways, you wouldn't like it, your babies—if they could still reckon— wouldn't like it, and we doctors would be sued off the face of the earth. Under proper circumstances, many women are being encouraged to try a vaginal delivery after a section and this procedure will eventually result in a small decline in the section rate. But we need never to go back to the traumatic vaginal delivery as a substitute for modern cesarian sections.

○○○○○○○

Toward decreasing infant mortality:

Efforts to decrease infant mortality in the United States have been directed largely from our nation's capitol, Washington, D.C.—and directed largely toward the rural South where the highest rate of infant mortality has historically been found. Many federal agencies and the Congress itself have directed legislation and efforts to bring down our embarrassingly high infant mortality. We are, after all, only fourteenth in the world in fetal survival and well behind all other developed nations and *we are not gaining.*

Most recently, a powerful private coalition has been formed to attack this national problem. Based in Washington, D.C., and called the Healthy Mothers, Healthy Babies Coalition, it boasts representation from seventy-five nationwide organizations, sixty state coalitions, and from all the federal agencies involved in the drive to reduce infant loss. This includes divisions of the National Institutes of Health, the U.S. Public Health Service, the Health Care Financing Administration, the Institutions of Medicine, and so on. It also includes the Washington-headquartered American College of Obstetricians and Gynecologists.

Important medical schools in the Washington, D.C., area are among the leaders in studying infant mortality and the chairman of one of these medical schools' department of obstetrics and gynecology is editor of the most widely read contemporary journal on advances in our specialty.

As a result of these multipronged Washington, D.C.–based efforts, infant mortality is steadily declining in our nation—even in the South.

Although prenatal care is now available across the nation, it is not available in the inner core of our major cities. Ironically, while infant mortality decreased throughout the nation in 1984, it *increased* by 16.5 percent in Washington, D.C.

○ ○ ○ ○ ○ ○ ○ ○ ○ ○ ○ ○ ○ ○ ○ ○ ○ ○ ○ ○ ○ ○ ○ ○ ○ ○ ○ ○ ○ ○ ○ ○ ○ ○ ○ ○ ○ ○ ○ ○ ○ ○ ○ ○ ○

# ∘5∘

# Giving Birth

## GOING TO THE HOSPITAL

There are a number of events that may bring you to the hospital while you are pregnant: prenatal classes, stress and non-stress testing, threatened abortion or premature labor, control of hypertension or of diabetes, and on and on. As you reach full term, you may be admitted to the hospital early one morning for induction of labor or for cesarian section if either of these procedures are indicated. You will certainly come to the hospital if your membranes rupture prematurely and, finally, you will certainly come when you are in labor.

Whatever brings you to the hospital, you will find a more relaxed birthing suite awaiting you. In the past, for a variety of reasons, labor and delivery areas were very structured and isolated. The more relaxed atmosphere of today allows for family-centered care and considerable visitation. You may already be aware of this from previous obstetrical experiences or from your prenatal classes. No matter. The atmosphere is much more like a pavilion in the park than a wing in a hospital.

Even so, there are some routines that must be followed:

- Hospital registration must take place with its long question-and-answer format. This step can be preempted at most hospitals by preregistering sometime during pregnancy. Ask your obstetrician.

- You must bring some things:
  - personal robe, gown, and slippers
  - personal toilet articles
  - a bed jacket and nursing bra
  - notepaper and pen
  - some clothing to bring home your baby in

- You must leave at home:
  - your jewelry and watch
  - your wallet and checkbook
  - personal linens, bath towels, etc. You may bring and use a satin pillow slip for your hair's sake if you wish.

- Remove heavy makeup, false eyelashes, contacts, and chewing gum.

Here are some questions you may need to be able to answer at the hospital. Be prepared:

- Your due date.

- Your previous obstetrical history.

- Any complications of this pregnancy.

- The name of your doctor and pediatrician.

- Your blood type and Rh factor.

- About the present labor—have membranes ruptured and when? Have contractions started and their characteristics? Any bleeding?

- Fetal activity and movement.

- Last food—what and how long ago?

- Disposition of contact lenses, jewelry, dental bridges or plates, gum.

- Any known allergies.

- Who is the closest responsible person right now?

Most always hospitals have an updated copy of your obstetrician's records and much of the information they need can be found in these records. Nevertheless, you should be able to answer most of the questions they ask you.

# INDUCTION OF LABOR

Sometimes it is wise and sometimes it is convenient to induce the natural phenomenon of labor. It is wise when certain conditions of mother or infant dictate that the uterus should be emptied. We have seen that much already in our talk on postmaturity (see pages 135–36). At other times, even long before full term (let alone postmaturity) it makes good sense to empty the uterus. For instance, severe diabetes, uncontrollable hypertension of pregnancy, or advancing Rh incompatibility could indicate early uterine evacuation. Under these circumstances, the only final decision would be how best to evacuate the uterus. Sometimes a section might be safer than an induction of labor. Faced with such a dilemma, you and your obstetrician would have to settle the issue, but many times induction of labor followed by vaginal delivery can safely accomplish all our goals.

Yes, and sometimes it is convenient to induce labor—the so-called elective induction of labor. It may be convenient for the obstetrician, but it may also be convenient for a mother who labors rapidly, lives far from the hospital, or who has responsibilities at home that are not easy to meet on an emergency basis. Whatever the reasons for an elective induction of labor, certain criteria must be met.

- There must be no question that the pregnancy is at full term.
- The baby must present as a vertex (head) and it must be within the deep true pelvis.
- The cervix must be soft, somewhat open, and favorable for induction.

Given all the above conditions, the elective induction of labor, properly monitored and carried out, is as safe—or safer—than normal labor. Many thousands of elective labor inductions attest to that fact.

Here's how induction of labor is carried out:

- Inductions are planned and thus the stomach and bowels are emptied by one means or another.
- An intravenous line is established and through it fluids and medications may be administered until well after deliv-

ery. Also—and most importantly—pitocin, the drug that initiates labor, is fed into the line by an electronic meter which gauges with great accuracy the amount delivered each minute.

An IV (intravenous line) has many advantages, and you can move, sit up, and even walk with an IV in place. No needle is involved after the first puncture. Besides supplying instant access to your system should that become necessary, it also avoids repeated needle punctures and keeps you hydrated, nourished, and electrolyte balanced. Little or no risk and superb advantages are common to all modern IV lines.

○ Monitoring of the fetal heart and the maternal uterine contractions is instituted. (See pages 261–70.)

○ The flow rate of pitocin is adjusted till regular uterine contractions are established with complete and adequate relaxations between them.

○ Most often the membranes will be artificially ruptured by your doctor provided that the presenting head is engaged within the pelvis and delivery is very likely within several hours. This should always be true with elective inductions. Indicated inductions are not always simple and may have to be repeated once or twice. Thus, the membranes may not always be ruptured in such cases until progressive labor is established for certain.

Induced labor usually proceeds quite briskly. The pitocin may be cut back or even be discontinued once the uterus begins to act on its own. Labor and fetal and maternal well-being must be monitored closely and constantly.

## Induction of labor by breast stimulation

It has long been known that stimulation of the nipples will produce uterine contractions. This fact is used as the basis for the breast stimulation test (BST), which serves as a guide for fetal health just as the usual pitocin stress test does, over which a BST has some advantages (see BST, page 269).

Using this stimulating principle, some clinics are actually inducing labor by breast stimulation techniques and are reporting satisfactory results. There will be more to report on this in future editions.

## LABOR

In 1969, Neil Armstrong, speaking from the moon, uttered his great observation which said in part, "One giant step for mankind." Few statements that I can recall have been able to compress so much of complex human endeavor so well. It ranks with Churchill's "Never in the history of human endeavor has so much been owed by so many to so few."

Great as these proclamations of our mortal achievement may be, they are eminently surpassed by the single, simple, small, and unassuming word *labor,* particularly when the word applies to women bringing forth and multiplying. From the very beginning of human events—however that was achieved—labor has preoccupied not only the laboring woman but has equally been the vector of social, political, medical, moral, familial, historical, and cultural evolution of all societies, wild or civilized. More has been recorded both in fact and fantasy about labor than any other human act, including the one that precedes it by some nine months. What can I add here? Only a short summary of the actual events as they transpire while labor unfolds:

### The onset

Labor usually begins in one of three ways:

° A bloody show. This is a vaginal secretion consisting of small amounts of blood and mucous. Bleeding in excess of a light period, however, is abnormal and should be reported. Sometimes you may spot for several hours after your doctor has performed a pelvic examination and such bleeding should not be considered as a show.

° Rupture of the membranes. This event should not be considered abnormal at full term and it may precede the onset of uterine contractions by several hours. It may, however, be a cause of concern if:

Your baby is not presenting normally. Your doctor will quite likely have informed you of this complication during an office visit and asked you to call at once if you suspect your membranes have ruptured.

The amniotic fluid that escapes is not clear. The presence of discoloration may indicate fetal distress and it rates action at once.

You should call your doctor if you believe that membranes have ruptured and you should stop eating. Rupture may be accompanied by a large volume of amniotic fluid, leaving no doubt in your mind what has happened. On the other hand, it may consist of a light but persistent trickle that just dampens your panties, your leg, or your bed linen. When in doubt, call.

° Uterine contractions. This is what labor is all about. As you already know, your uterus has been contracting regularly throughout most of your pregnancy. It simply contracts and relaxes on a more or less regular cycle and such contractions are usually quite painless, although you can feel your tummy knot up or harden. At the onset of labor, the contraction pattern changes. Instead of relaxing completely at the end of a contraction, uterine muscle now shortens a little bit with each new impulse. Thus, the uterine volume gradually diminishes, forcing the baby to go somewhere else to live. Diminished uterine volume forces the cervix to dilate and vaginal expulsion follows.

Contraction patterns may vary widely. Usually, though, they begin to be noticeable at twenty-to-thirty-minute intervals, lasting thirty to forty seconds. Gradually the interval closes, and in advanced labor, contractions are only a few minutes apart and may last somewhat longer.

How long? First labors are usually the longest and the intervals generally decrease as the number of pregnancies increases. Although there are wide variations, first labors generally terminate after twelve to fourteen hours, and on average, those that follow, after six to eight hours. These are all normal circumstance labors, mind you. Primelife mothers having their first baby tend to take a little longer. Many other factors influence the duration of labor including cervical softness and thickness, the strength of contractions, medications, abnormal presentations, pelvic size, and so forth. Read on.

## The division of labor

Human labor is divided into three stages as follows:

○ Stage One. The longest, it begins with the onset of progressive labor as the cervix begins to dilate and ends when the cervix is fully dilated. At this point your examiner states that the amount of dilation is ten centimeters, an approximation which may be mathematically true but which really means to all that the cervix is fully dilated (complete, in obstetrical parlance) and out of the baby's way. Labor may begin with the cervix almost closed (1 cm) or as much as three or more centimeters dilated. Moreover, the cervix may start out paper-thin and soft or it may be hard and long, an unpopular situation. Attempts to push down or bear down before full cervical dilation are useless and may be injurious because, until the cervix is completely gone, the baby can't get out of the uterus any more than a head of lettuce can be forced into those damnable plastic grocery bags.

○ Stage Two. The cervix no longer restrains the baby and active maternal bearing down, voluntary or reflex, pushes it out into the world. This stage of labor may last a few minutes or several hours, depending on many variables. Anesthesia, tight pelvic fits, first labors, lack of preparedness, and fear tend to slow things down. Previous labors and total relaxation tend to speed things up. Without anesthesia, there is an intense urge to bear down at this time and the urge should be answered. With anesthesia, particularly an epidural, such an urge is not felt and coaching is often necessary as contractions appear on the monitor screen.

○ Stage Three. The placenta separates and is expelled during this stage which usually lasts a few minutes but in rare instances may take much longer. A very uncommon condition unfolds when the placenta refuses to separate and cannot be separated manually by the doctor. Called placenta accreta, this very rare condition calls for prompt surgical treatment.

Most often, however, the placenta separates and comes

away quite promptly. Some physicians remove the placenta manually if spontaneous separation does not take place within a few minutes. This approach is quite safe in expert hands. At the same time the physician explores the uterus and cervix to make sure no hidden tears have taken place. Fetal blood is usually taken from the placental vessels and sent to the laboratory for a number of blood tests. These may include blood type and Rh, and serum tests for certain infections and for blood gas determinations.

And your baby now rests on your abdomen, you address one another, look at one another eye to eye—and you are on your own.

## False labor

Painless, more or less regular uterine contractions continue throughout most of all pregnancies. You already know this, but it is worth reminding you again. However, painful regular contractions may supervene at any time and when that happens, it is often difficult to tell whether labor has begun or whether false labor is paying a visit. Both mother and obstetrician can be fooled. The contractions are, after all, regular and they are painful. Here are some ways of telling the difference:

o The contractions. Generally the contraction frequency in false labor remains unchanged. If pains start out at, say, five-minute intervals, then that's the way they stay. In true labor, the intervals close regularly.

o The duration. After a period of several hours, false labor generally withers away—maybe to return later, maybe not. True labor is relentless and continues on.

o The company. False labor is not accompanied by bloody show (unless you have been examined internally), nor is it accompanied by membrane rupture—ever.

o The examination. Dilation or effacement (thinning) of the cervix does not take place under observation unless the labor is real. Further, it is becoming evident that fetal breathing diminishes sharply during real labor. Ultrasound examination can confirm this last point.

○ Mild sedation will usually stop false labor, and although alcohol is not safe in early pregnancy, a few ounces of sherry as term approaches often arrests false labor without doing any harm whatsoever. Wine is not to be used on a regular basis to prevent false labor. That's rationalizing.

Should you be subject to episodes of confirmed false labor, rest and/or diversionary tactics are helpful in driving the contractions away. Sedation or wine should be used only sparingly and infrequently.

In spite of the differences between true and false labor, it is sometimes almost impossible to differentiate the two conditions and observation in the hospital may become a necessary step. The important thing here is that the doctor must be sure that true but obstructed labor is not being overlooked.

Primelife mothers are no more prone to false labor than any other pregnant women.

## Prolonged labor

Not too long ago, prolonged labor was identified as any labor lasting over twenty-four hours in a first pregnancy or over fourteen hours in all subsequent pregnancies. These guidelines are no longer followed precisely and a further briefing on progressive labor is now necessary. The definition of labor stages noted on pages 155–56 still holds and the first stage of labor does consist of progressive cervical dilation along with continuous descent of the fetal presenting part, and the second stage consists of continuing descent of the fetus until delivery is achieved. Obstetricians following labor today, however, generally make further division in progressive labor activity in order to detect as early as possible what may become prolonged labor. Thus, there is described a latent and an active phase of cervical dilation, each with different rates of dilation. Also described separately is the rate of fetal descent, and a protracted descent rate is predictive of prolonged labor, as are abnormalities of the latent and active cervical curves.

So it becomes more complicated as we chop into segments the continuous process of labor in order to try and interpret its progress more efficiently. And it also becomes more difficult to tell you in hours what truly constitutes prolonged labor. Most likely all first labors terminate before twenty-four hours and all following labors within fourteen hours.

The techniques described above allow more rapid identification of what is likely to become prolonged labor and so allow for earlier intervention to correct whatever has gone wrong, which is usually one or any combination of the following:

° The passage. Certain variations in maternal bone structure or in soft tissues may make progressive labor difficult. It is usually possible to delineate these conditions by pelvic examination, but sometimes x-rays or ultrasound are needed for confirmation. Many of the changes are subtle and not easy to pick up by any method except observed labor.

° The passenger. An unusually large fetal head or any abnormal presentation of its body may also slow or obstruct the labor process. Even an average head may cause trouble if it does not come into the pelvis well flexed and facing down. These unusual fetal attitudes are detected by vaginal examinations during labor, occasionally assisted by x-rays or ultrasound.

° The powers. Uterine contractions with ever-diminishing uterine volume are the propelling force. Usually it is a very sufficient energy source. Sometimes it is not. Pain relief methods may interfere with uterine muscle activity. So may uterine overdistention (large or multiple fetuses), fear, multiparity (many pregnancies), exhaustion, and yes, primelife, too, although not very often.

Once the diagnosis of prolonged or potentially prolonged labor has been made, treatment is instituted. Such treatment may be rest, followed by pitocin augmentation, it may be cesarian section, or it may be a change in the pain relief patterns. Each prolonged pattern is dealt with on an individual basis to assure a safe and successful outcome. No primelife mother will be in *true* labor and undelivered for days and days. That simply doesn't happen anymore.

### The labor and delivery suite—you have arrived

Some of this information is old hat already, but it is a good time to review what happens once you enter the hallowed halls where you will be unburdened. After the routine admission information has been obtained and your obstetrician notified, you may be subject to several indignities.

o Enemas. Only your own doctor can order this procedure. All inquiries should be routed in that direction. Enemas are sometimes withheld if labor is advancing rapidly and if certain complications exist. Usually, though, enemas clear the lower bowel and make later stages of labor more comfortable and less embarrassing for you. If all things are normal, you can take an enema at home.

o Perineal shaves. You can do this at home too if you can see or if you have a helping partner. Sometimes shaving of the perineal area is delayed until you reach the point of delivery. Sometimes the shave simply does not take place, particularly if you are not having an episiotomy (see below).

o Intravenous lines. Some mothers object to intravenous fluid and electrolyte support during labor, but by and large, an open vein with fluids running is a marvelous and protective channel throughout labor and delivery. The earlier section on labor induction recites the many advantages of intravenous support. Again, there is no significant danger involved, movement about the labor suite is not inhibited, and it stands ready to receive instant medication should you or yours need it for any reason. Do not try to avoid this important step.

o Standard procedures. You will of course have standard vital signs taken and recorded. Temperature, pulse, respirations, and blood pressure are vital baseline observations as are fetal heart tones and uterine contraction rates. A nurse, resident, intern, or your doctor will examine you internally to determine if membranes are ruptured, the presentation of your baby, and the degree of dilation and effacement of your cervix. Routine blood and urine samples are obtained, and that's about it.

And so to bed. Now bed may be just that—a bed in a routine labor room. It may also be a brass bed in a birthing room, which is prepared for labor, delivery, and recovery. That takes a very special brass bed, but they are making them now. Bed may also be a reclining chair if you are going to use the now popular chair delivery method. Whatever—unless your obstetrician sends you out in the halls to walk—you recline in some sort of reclining apparatus while life unfolds. And you and your baby will most likely be monitored.

## MONITORED LABOR

Time was when monitoring of labor consisted of a friendly hand on the abdomen to feel for contractions along with an occasional stethoscope to listen for fetal heart tones. Those casual days are mostly gone and labor surveillance has been delivered into the hands of microchips, video displays, and computer alarm systems.

Electronic labor monitors are elegant devices which, when properly placed on the abdomen (external) or in the uterus (internal), more or less faithfully record uterine contractions and fetal heart rates. External monitoring is safe and painless. Internal monitoring may cause some discomfort while being introduced and carries a slight risk. Both methods are described in the technical section in detail (pages 261–70). The video display of uterine contractions and fetal heart rates allows real-time observation of labor and its effect on the fetal heart and for early intervention should fetal distress develop. It also provides a permanent record of labor events.

Some things need to be pointed out here:

° Electronic monitoring is not perfect. Should the sensing devices not be applied correctly and remain in place, or should they be defective even temporarily, the information they provide will not be reliable.

° The information that monitors provide must be interpreted. This whole process is still really in its infancy and, while certain basic abnormalities are clearly established, there is still much divergence of opinion in certain abnormal states. Some monitors are computer scanned and sound an alarm if an abnormal pattern is recognized. That pattern *still* must be viewed by a humanoid for a final interpretation.

° A number of obstetricians feel that routine electronic monitoring has increased the cesarian section rate without increasing fetal well-being. Others feel that the procedure is indispensable in modern obstetrical management. Again, it is in its infancy and these conflicts will eventually be resolved. No matter what the resolution, monitoring will persist.

o As a primelife mother, you will more than likely have a monitored labor. It may restrict you to a bed, chaise, or recliner environment, but don't fight it. The weight of current evidence indicates that such surveillance of your labor is a safe, valuable, and thoroughly fascinating way to watch your labor unfold.

Again, monitoring methods along with sample tracings are reviewed in depth starting on page 261.

### ANESTHESIA

An old Episcopal prayer offered in church until recently following the successful delivery of a communicant mother went partly thus: "O Almighty God, we give thee humble thanks for that thou hast been graciously pleased to preserve through the great pain and peril of childbirth, this woman, thy servant. . . ."

Well, all that prose makes marvelous, if chilling, liturgical syntax, but listen—so many Episcopal obstetricians objected to the prayer's wording that it has fallen into disfavor and is seldom used anymore. Primelife mothers who take good care of themselves are not, after all, likely to be in great peril during childbirth, at least not once they are safely driven to the hospital. Similarly, they are not likely to be in any great pain during childbirth.

Hold on, now. Don't jump the gun. No one—least of all me—is suggesting that pain is not a part of childbearing. Far from it. Labor and delivery left to itself can be torture *under some circumstances.* One does not have to be pregnant, to labor, or to deliver—or even be a woman—to testify to that fact. I for one can and will. But present-day pain relief procedures safely bypass most of the discomfort attendant upon the birth process.

Here are some thoughts about pain and childbearing: The degree of pain felt by different individuals submitting to identical pain stimulation varies greatly. There are at least two components here:

○ Individual pain thresholds vary. Gateways for pain sensation vary widely and can be consciously closed by certain individuals.

○ Fear. Fear of pain and the certainty that it is going to be experienced mounts a reaction that can triple the pain that is sensed, as well as provoking a number of strange responses. An old obstetrician that I knew used to perform the following incredible procedure to stop vomiting of pregnancy when *all else* failed. Into his patients' bedroom (obstetricians used to make house calls!) he would visibly bring a red-hot poker. At the same time a family accomplice would sneak in a piece of meat and an icicle (this only worked in the winter and up north when icicles were available). Shielding the poor pregnant vomiter's abdomen from her, he would indicate that the red-hot poker would be laid across her belly and would stop the vomiting! And so the poker fell on the meat and the icicle on her tummy! Most mothers stopped vomiting. It's amazing that they didn't miscarry. It's also amazing what used to be done in the name of medicine! Now, that story is mostly true, but it belongs in the realm of the distant past. Still, no one could tell that unfortunate mother that she did not feel herself being branded and smell her flesh as it broiled. And her vomiting may have been cured— and someone else had a rare steak dinner.

Present-day prenatal instructions in the process of labor and delivery can largely dispel fear, particularly fear of the unknown, and such instruction can also provide insight into methods of nerve-impulse gate closing so as to reduce pain stimulation reaching sensory centers. Despite all this, some prolonged and obstructed labors can be very painful without help.

There is virtually no reason for a primelife mother to refuse pain relief during labor or to feel guilty about receiving it. Moreover, there is virtually no reason for anyone to withold pain relief from you.

Attempts to reduce the pain of birth are as old as pain and birth. In America, it was bite the bullet or drink some whiskey until twilight sleep was introduced early this century. To induce this sleep, combinations of morphine and scopolamine were given until sweet oblivion was reached. Such medications were depressing to the fetus, but very acceptable to laboring mothers. Resuscitative techniques generally protected the infants.

Twilight sleep has largely been discarded in this country. However, moderate amounts of narcotics and other supportive drugs are still often given in early labor until more definitive anesthesia may be introduced. The amounts that are given are not sufficient to produce fetal respiratory depression and usually disappear from the circulation before delivery occurs. Such agents produce analgesia or partial pain relief. Anesthesia, on the other hand, usually produces complete pain relief.

## General anesthesia

Scotland, the hallowed birthplace of Scotch—a great general anesthetic itself—was also the birthplace of inhalation anesthesia for obstetrical purposes. Sir James Simpson began using ether to comfort patients while they gave birth. Queen Victoria heard of all this and fetched him to Buckingham Palace to attend upon and ease the birth of her son, Edward. Inhalation anesthesia spread rapidly to other countries and was first used in the United States in Boston. It is not known whether it was first used on a Lodge or a Cabot. But that's where it started.

Today, general anesthesia still has a place in obstetrical management. The agents may be given intravenously (pentothal, for instance) or by inhalation (nitrous oxide, ether, or others), but the end result is complete sleep and complete dependency upon the anesthetist. What must be considered about a general anesthetic?

○ General anesthesia is an important part of our armamentarium. With it we can very quickly induce sleep and sometimes that is very important. If, for example, a mother is bleeding excessively from a separated placenta, if an umbilical cord is down, if convulsions are occurring, if instant sleep is needed for any reason, general anesthesia is the way to go.

○ It is true that general agents get into the fetal circulation very quickly and can put the baby to sleep along with its mother. This risk must be tolerated when general anesthesia is indicated. Modern methods of resuscitation can protect newborns who are asleep.

° One very significant problem with general anesthesia is the fact that most obstetrical patients are poorly prepared to go to sleep. Mainly this is because their stomachs are usually not empty. Even if no food has been ingested for many hours, old food tends to stay in a full-term mother's stomach for very long periods of time, and almost always under a general anesthetic, vomiting will occur. Thus, it is important—more important than almost any other advice I can give you—not to eat or drink if you feel that you may be starting labor. You may never need to be put to sleep but you also want to wake up healthy afterward.

## Conduction anesthesia

When nerve impulses from hurting tissue are blocked and prevented from moving on up to the brain, we have induced conduction anesthesia. Regardless of the many conduction techniques involved, the agents used are all derived from the cocaine family of drugs. Cocaine, made from the leaves of the coca bush, has been used in South America for centuries to relieve pain of all sorts, physical and spiritual. The leaves were simply chewed to release the potent and habituating drug.

Although spinal anesthesia with cocaine was reported over 100 years ago, the first real research into the clinical use of the drug was conducted in this country early in this century by a famous surgeon who accidentally became the first American cocaine addict. Before his death, his contributions to pain relief and to surgery were enormous.

The basic nuclear structure of cocaine provides the core for all modern conduction anesthetics, and at last count there were over sixteen of them in active use, each with a specific indication.

Here are the common conduction anesthetic routes:

° Local. Given directly into a local painful or soon-to-be-painful body area, anesthesia is achieved promptly and lasts up to an hour. If allergies are eliminated, it is a very safe way to relieve pain. It is useful during delivery when an episiotomy is to be made and the mother wishes minimal pain relief.

° Local block. The same or a similar agent as that used for local infiltration is now used to block nerve trunks that supply tissues slightly removed from the location of the block. Thus, a pudendal block is infiltrated around the pudendal nerves as they approach the vagina and its entrance. Thus, not only can an episiotomy be established with comfort, but the pain of vaginal stretching is reduced. This block is given just a few moments before delivery and, as with a simple local, this is a very safe procedure in the absence of novocaine and related drug allergies.

A paracervical block is given through the back of the vagina into nerve plexuses around the base of the cervix. It takes some minutes to be effective and, when working well, allows the use of outlet forceps as well as an episiotomy, with some comfort. This block can initiate serious complications, mainly fetal. At least 25 percent of paracervical blocks produce significant fetal heart decelerations, some of which may be responsible for mortal problems. This block therefore is still described, but seldom indicated or used anymore.

∘ Spinal blocks. In this very effective anesthetic, a needle is inserted through the backbone spaces and into the dura, a tough membrane which encases the spinal nerve cord and which contains spinal fluid. The anesthetic fluid is now injected directly into the dural space.

Spinal anesthetics have many advantages. They are swift and sure and produce as high or as low a level of anesthesia as desired. They can be used for a vaginal or a cesarian birth equally well. They are, however, not without serious problems. One must first be certain that there are no allergies to novocaine and related drugs and further, blood pressure, which becomes very unstable, must be monitored constantly along with other vital signs. The most common adverse spinal reaction is the postspinal headache occurring in 1 to 2 percent of all spinals. Such headaches are very painful and may last many days, requiring rest flat in bed. This is no place for a primelife mother to be after delivery and so spinal anesthetics have limited use in regular obstetrics.

One example of its use is for precipitate delivery. Every so often a mother hits the doors of the labor suite in tumultuous labor, moving along faster than you can say Planned Parenthood. Such precipitous labor is often accompanied by very meaningful pain. It is also often accompanied by a mad dash to a delivery table with panties, slips, and shoes falling by the wayside and attendants opening up delivery equipment faster than your child is going to open up its Christmas presents when it is four.

Such labors are often preceded by a hearty meal which still lies mainly within the stomach. So, all taken together, we need quick pain relief without the danger of food aspiration. Here a spinal is virtually perfect. But there are other indications as well.

° Continuous epidural block. This is the technique which seems to best meet the needs of mother, fetus, and obstetrician. Women not wishing to avoid pain relief completely still wish to be conscious and alert during labor and delivery. Continuous epidural blocks allow this to happen in comfort.

Here is more about this method:

° An epidural is administered much like a spinal, but the dural membrane is *not* pierced, thus the word *epidural.* A needle is placed in the epidural space and through it a fine plastic catheter is inserted and the needle withdrawn. This catheter may be put in place very early in labor in anticipation of discomfort as labor progresses. It does not impede movement and patients can lie about or sit up any way they choose. Whenever the anesthesia is to be started, a test dose is administered through the catheter to observe for any unusual reaction and to make certain of the location of the catheter tip. If all is satisfactory, a full anesthetic dose is then delivered.

° Anesthesia can be added regularly throughout labor as needed and may be continued for many hours with safety. During this time, of course, vital maternal signs are monitored regularly, along with evidence of fetal well-being.

° The mother will probably lie on her left side after an anesthetic level is achieved. This, as always, is to keep pressure off the major blood vessels which supply the uterus and therefore the fetus. Also she may be asked to breathe oxygen for a while if her blood pressure takes a transient drop. This is to assure that plenty of oxygen arrives at the uterus.

○ Epidural anesthesia is always preceded by a venous line and often by a fast-running IV solution. Thus proper hydration and blood volume is assured from the beginning. Further, the IV is instantly available for the use of supportive medications—something you already know about.

○ Labor is usually not altered in any serious way by epidurals. Sometimes it slows down temporarily, but often it is enhanced by the relaxation that accompanies pain relief so that labor speeds up. Low outlet forceps may need to be used at the point of delivery since the intense urge to bear down has been temporarily obliterated. Coaching may help to overcome this and often mother can watch through mirrors and see when she is pushing down effectively.

## EPISIOTOMY

An episiotomy is a clean surgical incision made just at the time of delivery. It is either directed straight from the vagina toward the rectum (median episiotomy) or laterally to one side of the rectum (mediolateral episiotomy). The direction that the incision takes depends upon the amount of room available between the vagina and the rectum and the amount of room needed. Both variables vary. That is, the distance between the vagina and rectum is not constant in all women and the amount of room needed depends upon the baby's size and presentation, and moreover, what intravaginal manipulations may be necessary to deliver it properly.

Episiotomies never used to be done. They are entirely the result of male intervention into the birth process, and willingly, I freely confess to being a participant in this intervention. In order to prevent some of the horrid tears into the rectum and adjacent tissues that they had seen (once allowed into the birth rooms), male physicians began making straight incisions to avoid such tears and to make repair much more straightforward after delivery. This *almost* routine practice has persisted and the majority of deliveries managed by obstetricians of *both* sexes are still accompanied by an episiotomy. However, consumerism, good or bad, has entered into this very private anatomical arena too. A measurable number of people both in the profession and out feel that episiotomies are unnecessary, do not spare tissue, increase recovery time and postpartum discomfort, and do not accomplish the things they are supposed to accomplish.

It is hard for one mother to assess the validity of these statements. She cannot, after all, retrace her steps and do without an episiotomy if she has had one and vice versa. She may have sustained an episiotomy in her first pregnancy with healing discomfort afterward, then had no episiotomy with her second and felt no postpartum discomfort at all. Thus, it appears to follow to her, at least, that the first delivery would have been easier for her afterward without an episiotomy. If your obstetrician, whom you trust, feels an episiotomy is necessary, let her do it.

Here are a few more things about an episiotomy:

° Complications from episiotomies are unusual. They can break down, get hematomas (blood clots), bleed, and get infected. So can tears. Even the best of them can extend on into the rectum and other tissues, requiring skilled repairs, but not as skilled as tears require for correction. Very rarely, prolonged discomfort follows an episiotomy and is most evident at period time.

° Episiotomy repairs generally restore almost normal vaginal anatomy following a delivery, although they cannot totally prevent stretching of the tissues which support the bladder and the rectum. However, the tone and size of the vaginal barrel is much better supported by an episiotomy repair and this can have important sexual overtones. A very loose vaginal entrance and barrel can and often does reduce sensation for both partners. This is extremely well documented. Those opposed to episiotomies hold that such lost sexual pleasure may thus be enhanced elsewhere. Where?

° There should be no such thing as a routine episiotomy. The only thing that should be routine in life is going to bed at night—and even that will soon be denied you as it has been denied me for thirty years. But to return—episiotomies are only to be done on indication, not routinely.

° The suture material used to reconstruct an episiotomy is absorbable and removal of stitches is thus avoided. Since some of the sutures are running, as in hemming, and some are interrupted, as in trussing, it is almost impossible to keep track of the number of stitches involved in any one repair. If your obstetrician says 200, then you have been repaired. If she says 5, you have been trussed. But no one would do that to you.

## FORCEPS

Forceps are like a pair of tongs that can be separated into individual arms at their fulcrum. Thus, each arm may be introduced into the vagina separately and rejoined at the fulcrum. Properly applied, they surround the baby's head and can turn it or extract it as need may be. It is altogether likely that crude forceps were used in ancient cultures and died with those cultures.

As the world awakened from the Middle Ages, medicine flourished and medical men began to exert pressure to learn more about pregnancy, labor, and delivery. This was felt to be very improper and they were systematically excluded from the birthing chambers. One resourceful Dutch physician dressed as a woman and actually got in to observe a delivery. He was discovered, of course, and for his pains was burned to death. Much later, another Dutch physician, Dr. William Chamberlain, having learned some basic anatomy and not wanting to get burned, reinvented the forceps—crude wooden tongs covered with leather. Midwives began calling upon him in cases of prolonged obstructed labor after quilling the patient's nose with feathers or stuffing it (the nose) with snuff—all to induce protracted sneezing—failed to effect delivery. Many times, Dr. Chamberlain was able to deliver such tortured women and gradually his reputation grew. So did the envy of other physicians and the coveting of his secret instrument, for he had told no one about it and did not publish any of his methods. Long after he was gone the secret was still held within his family as his sons continued his medical practice. Finally, one of them, in a moment of financial embarrassment, agreed to sell the forceps secret. But he only revealed one arm of the forceps! Nevertheless, it was many years before the buyers realized they had been had. That tells us something.

And that's how the story of modern obstetric forceps began. Over the intervening years, the types of forceps multiplied to respond to all sorts of delivery problems and they became very sophisticated metal instruments of which the profession was very proud (I have a very beautiful pair of gold forceps given to me many years ago, but now retired to a shadow box on my study wall). Before we move on to the present-day use of forceps, let me point out a few facts, now forgotten.

Remember that before forceps, prolonged obstructed labor often spelled death for both mother and child. There was no way to get the baby out. Cesarian section, usually performed at the point of maternal death, often did not even save the child and so such a dreadful operation was usually an agonal decision when all hope was gone.

Once the forceps concept caught on, all sorts of them were invented to manage particular vaginal delivery problems. One was for turning the baby's head, one for the after-coming breech head, one for transverse positions of the head, even one to crush the infant's head like a nut so it would come through the pelvis! Anything, anything to effect a vaginal delivery and avoid the deadly cesarian section.

Three basic forceps applications were recognized:

○ High. The presenting head was not even in the pelvis and the forceps application had to be made far up in the uterus. Only very skilled operators could do this and it has long since disappeared into history.

○ Mid. In this situation, the head is stationed about half-way through the pelvis and, generally, in an abnormal position—either turned sideways or posterior. Midforceps, then, generally consist of applying the forceps, turning the child's head to the proper position, and then pulling it out. The indication for midforceps is obstructed labor with the head arresting in the midpelvis. Such forceps application require skill and experience, and today the procedure is less and less commonly used. Why? Because the cesarian section has become a very safe operation and is considered less damaging to both mother and child than most midforceps application.

○ Low or outlet. In this situation the presenting head is very nearly ready to deliver and is in proper position and alignment in the pelvis. Such forceps applications are used to assist in the terminal delivery process when mother may be exhausted or when, because of a block anesthetic, she cannot marshal the expulsive forces needed to deliver her baby. Low forceps are safe, simple, and still often done today. There is no real evidence of maternal or fetal damage because of them.

So it becomes clear, then, that the outlet forceps application is just about its only use today. Thus, all the fancy forceps of the past are in museums or shadow boxes, not delivery suites. And it is a good thing.

But remember this clearly: Obstructed labor still takes place with about the same frequency as always. However, it is being managed by cesarian section. Thus the section rate is climbing. But equally, the rate of dangerous operative vaginal deliveries is declining. Which would you prefer for yourself? And your child?

The modern use of low forceps is as follows:

o Adequate anesthesia is required. Sometimes a pudendal block is sufficient, but it is preferable to have a general, spinal, or epidural anesthetic in place.

o The presenting head must be deep in the pelvis and beyond all narrow potentially obstructing levels. Its crown may already be visible at the vaginal entrance.

o Most often, an episiotomy is a prerequisite to low forceps application. This is not universally true, however. Sometimes the vagina is very commodious after previous deliveries with or without episiotomies. Under these circumstances, an episiotomy may be avoided.

o When all is thus ready, the forceps are disengaged and each arm inserted separately into the vagina alongside the baby's head and then reengaged. Gentle traction pulls the head through the small remaining distance and delivery is initiated.

## VACUUM EXTRACTION

In recent times, some very clever and innovative obstetricians have developed a method of extracting babies which may be even safer than the low forceps procedure. Called a vacuum extractor, this instrument is nothing more than a very small, skillfully designed plumber's helper. It is placed against the fetal head, a vacuum is created, and extraction is then accomplished as with forceps—by pulling. Proponents say that this device is much less likely to compress fetal or maternal tissue and is thus the safest way to assist in a low situation delivery. There is ample evidence today to support their claim. Still not widely used, the technique is gaining more support as its equipment becomes more sophisticated and more evidence of its safety is generated.

## GRAVITY–PARITY

In obstetrics, gravity has nothing to do with the attraction of earth and parity has nothing to do with the American dollar's stand against foreign currency. So here are the real meanings.

When a woman becomes pregnant, she is gravid (Latin: *gravidus,* "heavy, as with child"). The first time she is pregnant she is designated as primigravid or primigravida, the second, secunidigravida, and as more and more pregnancies unfold, multigravida. These pregnancies may end in normal term deliveries, abortions, premature labors, ectopics, or living or dead infants. No matter what the outcome, each time a woman is pregnant, gravida goes up one more notch.

Following a term delivery, she is now designated as parous (Latin: *parere,* "to bring forth"). Thus, a mother who is gravida 5, para (short for parous) 3 has been pregnant five times and has three living children. The other two pregnancies may have ended in abortion or ectopic or—get this now—she may be still carrying that fifth pregnancy. So you are gravida 1, para 0 while you are pregnant with your first child, and you are gravida 1, para 1 when that child is in your arms.

That is not very simple terminology, and I have not made it any simpler by trying to explain it. All I can say is if you are gravida 5, para 0, you are in trouble and if you are gravida 5, para 5, you are in even bigger trouble, and you don't need to be reading this.

# PRESENTATION AND POSITION

## Presentation

This term is used to identify what major part of the fetal anatomy presents at the pelvic entrance and thus how the baby really lies within the uterus. In the majority of instances, the head (vertex) is what presents and so this presentation is properly called vertex. Occasionally the baby's bottom is first into the pelvis and this is called a breech presentation. Most often, breech presentations are associated with twins or more, uterine malformations, abnormal placental location, and other disorders, but a breech may also just happen for no apparent reason.

Very rarely, presentation of such unusual anatomical areas as the shoulder, the back, or even multiple body parts may be encountered. Such uncommon presentations are usually treated by cesarian section, particularly if they are found to be present at full term.

## Position

Position describes how the presenting part actually lies. Thus, a vertex or head presentation may lie in six positions, all based on the location of the back of the baby's head (the occiput). The occiput may be forward, backward, or transverse in the maternal pelvis and in all those positions may lie on the right or left maternal side. Moreover, if the presenting head is poorly flexed, it may be lying in six positions of the forehead. Similarly, based on the location of its sacrum, a breech may also lie in at least six positions. And so the story becomes more and more complicated. You do not have to know or appreciate these variable positions, but your obstetrician does. At least now you may have some grasp of the terms *presentation* and *position*.

# MACROSOMIA

Obstetricians cannot simply call a big baby a big baby. That would be too simple and straightforward. Thus babes born weighing over 4,500 grams (10 pounds) are cleverly identified as macrosomic (big bodies—what else?). Macrosomia is identified with certain obstetrical problems.

○ It is often associated with diabetes, particularly poorly controlled diabetes. Further, maternal obesity, excessive pregnancy weight gain, postmaturity, and, alas, primelife pregnancy also share the association to a certain degree.

○ Quite understandably, cesarian section rates are very high in macrosomia (35 percent as a general rule) and vaginal delivery is fraught with difficulties, often centering upon delivery of the shoulders of all things.

○ Macrosomic infants are more likely to be male and are more likely to have some degree of birth trauma due to their large size.

Your obstetrician will follow you carefully for signs of excessive fetal size, but it is not always easy to determine this condition by examination or even by ultrasound.

## POSTPARTUM

A casual walk down the postpartum (after delivery) halls of a modern obstetrical hospital today is much like going to a local craft fair. Most doors are festooned with every manner of local creative artwork announcing the sex of the newborn child and adorned with every object that this child might possibly be interested in during its first ten years of life. Gone from the postpartum floors—mostly, thank goodness—are cigars of poor quality, foul odor, and banded with the newborn child's sex.

The mother who delivered in the fields and then continued her work has been the subject of great anecdotal storytelling. She probably existed, but that word also pretty well characterized her total life picture—*existed.* The opposite extreme was in vogue during the early part of this century when mothers were kept in the hospital for ten days and in bed for the first seven of those days following the most normal delivery. When they finally were allowed to get up, they often fainted and they felt very weak indeed, much like astronauts returning to earth and to gravity forces. Doctors said this weakness proved that the bed rest had been necessary! Not the first mistake we have made.

Well, today's hospital stay following delivery is a vastly different and shorter episode. So much is crammed into it that it is rarely boring and going home is somewhat like a parole. In the first place, if you have elected to try rooming in, your baby is with you most of the time. Moreover, in many hospitals your coconspirator is also allowed to room in and thus you have a "ménage à trois" with none of the advantages such an arrangement is touted to provide. With so much going on, with nursing personnel and doctors dropping in whenever for whatever, with meals coming in a different time warp and visitors coming during gas time, with all this and more, the hospital experience is best gotten behind you quickly. There are, however, some things you might want to know about it.

There are some sources of pain after delivery and some of them may get your attention rather forcibly for a while:

○ Episiotomy. Should you have had an episiotomy, the area surrounding it may be significantly swollen and tender. It still heals better than a tear. Most hospitals have sitz bath facilities and, as a rule, you can start them anytime you want to. Local medications can be prescribed by your obstetrician to help reduce the discomfort.

○ Hemorrhoids. Even if your episiotomy goes nowhere near the rectum, you can still develop significant rectal pain from hemorrhoids, even if you have never had such problems before. Straining down at the time of delivery may be the culprit that induces this problem. No matter what the cause, your bowels must be made to function fairly soon after delivery (within a day or so) or the situation gets worse. Local applications and creams help make life tolerable but you may get to have a close relationship with a rubber donut ring, the postpartum life belt.

○ Breasts. Almost at once after delivery, signals are sent to the breasts explaining the fact that a baby has been delivered and that they need to start making milk. Naturally, they respond and (usually within forty-eight hours) breast engorgement takes place. Engorgement is not due to milk itself, but to swelling of the glandular components of the breast as they prepare to make milk. It is only after such swelling subsides that true milk starts to flow. If you are nursing, the milk will flow and the discomfort leaves. If you do not plan to nurse, medications are given to you to inhibit breast engorgement and discomfort. No matter which route you plan to take, your breasts at this time should be very well supported by an appropriate bra.

  ○ Afterpains. Your uterus will continue to contract regularly after delivery in order to prevent abnormal bleeding and to help your uterus shrink to its normal size (involution). Such contractions are usually not painful after the first delivery. Subsequent deliveries, however, may be followed by painful contractions which are called afterpains. When that takes place, the discomfort is often accentuated by nursing since breast stimulation produces uterine contractions. (Remember BST?) The afterpain discomfort subsides in a few days.

Other concerns are:

  ○ Lochia. No matter whether you have had a normal vaginal delivery or a cesarian section, you will still have a vaginal discharge which is called lochia. At first bloody and fairly heavy, it soon decreases and within a week is a moderate blood-tinged discharge. You need a sanitary pad for some weeks, but you cannot use a vaginal tampon until you have been examined to confirm healing. That may take four to six weeks. Your lochia may continue that long, particularly if you are nursing. You may even have some bloody drainage off and on until your first period. You should report any unusual increase in vaginal bleeding or the presence of anything in your discharge that looks like tissue or is otherwise unusual to you.

  ○ The bladder. Being in close proximity with all that goes on during labor and delivery, your bladder is subject to some pressure, stretching, and other general indignities at that time. A catheter is generally inserted just before delivery to make sure that your bladder is empty and thus out of the way, both of harm and of delivery. Moreover, if labor is fairly long, your bladder may fill up and you may not be able to empty it yourself. Thus, to the catheter. Usually this situation happens after an epidural has already been put in place so catheter insertion is at least painless.

  Even after a normal delivery you may not be able to

urinate at first and a catheterization may be necessary. Done gently, the procedure may be somewhat unpleasant but only for a moment or so. Very occasionally, enough swelling of the urethra (bladder entrance) or enough stretching of the bladder walls results in complete urinary obstruction and it becomes necessary to have an indwelling catheter set in place. Usually called a Foley catheter, these devices are held in place by an inflatable rubber balloon and they are commonly left in for a day or so. No matter what, before very long you will be going normally, just like before.

Because of all these bladder items described above, infection (cystitis) is not an unusual postdelivery complication. It is characterized by frequent and painful, often bloody urination, and it may begin anywhere from a few hours to a few weeks after delivery. Fortunately, cystitis responds quickly to simple antibiotics.

° The blues. Don't let anyone kid you about the blues. It can happen to you, and be very upsetting and annoying when it does—and very real. Usually it spreads its wings of gloom a day or so after delivery. You may be the happiest, most fulfilled primelife woman in the world, but your moment of glory may dissolve into tears, tears you can't explain. So don't try to.

There are many theories about the postpartum blues, which means no one knows the real cause. The good news, though, is that the blues go away as quickly as they came, usually within a few days.

There is a serious emotional disorder that can follow delivery and must not be confused with the ordinary blues. This disorder is a true psychosis, and it is very rare and usually settles upon mothers with a previous and serious emotional disorder. Moreover, it tends to appear weeks or even months after delivery. It is so uncommon, I shouldn't even mention it. Don't worry about it. Stable is as stable does.

Clean up, paint up, fix up. During your hospital stay, your personal hygiene can proceed virtually unchanged. You cannot—and wouldn't want to—douche or use vaginal tampons. Otherwise, you can shower, bathe, shampoo, and make up in all your traditional paints—the armor of amour.

You can usually eat what you want to, if they have it. Some

hospitals are featuring gourmet meals and some even give you and father a special champagne dinner after delivery on the house. Check into that.

Following a normal delivery your hospital stay may be one day or several, depending on many factors. Your home situation, finances, recovery rate, baby's health, and other factors all enter into the leave-taking time. Don't push it too hard—you may miss the room service!

Your doctor or an associate, your baby's pediatrician, and the hospital nursing staff will all visit you daily. Write down the questions you want to ask any of them. That's why I told you to bring pen and paper.

Male baby circumcision is not done routinely anymore. Your pediatrician will discuss this with you and you will arrive at a decision based on the recommendations you get. Circumcision can be done almost anytime after a normal delivery, and for some reason that escapes me, doesn't seem to bother the little fellows very much.

Semiprivate rooms are often segregated, that is, smokers and nonsmokers are not integrated when possible. If you are still a smoker and happen to be sharing quarters with a nonsmoker, be kind and considerate. If you are a nonsmoker and get put in with a smoker, pitch a fit!

If you are Rh negative, be certain that Rh vaccine is given you if indicated. Almost never is this important step overlooked after delivery, but if you don't get it double-check. Remember, if your baby is Rh negative, you don't need vaccination.

And while speaking of vaccination, rubella (German measles) vaccine is often given postpartum to mothers who are shown by laboratory tests not to be immune. Lately this practice has been questioned by some investigators so you would have to discuss this with your own doctor.

If you have enjoyed good hospital care, let the staff know it by telling them or writing to administration, or both.


## RECOVERY FROM A SECTION

If you have had a section, you are now both postpartum and postoperative. Your recovery rate is thus somewhat slower and you may very well spend an extra day or two in the hospital. The things I am about to tell you vary from one hospital to another and not all sections are the same, much depending upon the conditions involved at the time of surgery. Thus, a recovery from a repeat cesarian section is likely to be much more rapid than from a section following a difficult labor or associated with hemorrhage or severe hypertension and other abnormal conditions.

Most often your first day is spent in bed with feeding being accomplished intravenously, at least for part of the day, and with a Foley (indwelling catheter) in your bladder. If all goes well, the IV and the catheter come out on day two and you join the upwardly mobile society—slowly. Oral feedings begin and progress to a regular diet as fast as tolerated, which, with some hospital foods, may take some time even in health. The next day is usually gas oriented. The sooner you eat, the sooner you get gas but the sooner it is over with. Finally, you will be able to expel gas and now an enema will be helpful.

You can shower and shampoo the second day if your doctor approves and if all is well. You are generally advised to stay out of the tub for a while, at least until your skin incision is well healed. Incidentally, some obstetricians use absorbable stitches that do not require removal. Some prefer to use clips or nonabsorbable sutures and either of those require removal on the fourth or fifth day.

Once all these matters are attended to and your bowels and bladder function as of old—well, almost of old—it is time to say farewell and strike out for home.

## AT HOME

Clearly, there are a great many variables in postpartum events and care. Much depends upon where you are in this country (or any country), what sort of labor and delivery you have had, and what personal management philosophies reside in your obstetrician's heart. Always remember, if you are in any doubt about what is going on, ask! But now you'd best be getting home.

Coming home is not simple for a number of reasons:

    &deg; There is no one to wait on you unless it is a relative who will also peer over you and give you advice.

○ Getting around may be more difficult than you thought.

○ You have a twenty-four-hour responsibility whose schedule doesn't always—in fact very seldom does—coincide with yours. This responsibility can be very demanding and can let its demands be known in a number of unpleasant ways.

○ The blues may still haunt you a bit but they will leave more quickly than any of the above.

○ The pecking order and the loving order may change somewhat—or appear to change—and this may not sit too well around the castle for a while.

○ If you leave the drawbridge down, your friends will come a-chittering and a-chattering to tell you what the matter is with you.

Life's order of importance of events has been in disarray for you for some time. At homecoming it is screwed up even worse. What is most important in your life now? A clean place? A clean baby's bottom? Bonding? Sex? Your career (which keeps calling)? Your detergent? Your relatives? The PTA? Your dance instructor? Your pediatrician? Your obstetrician (can't remember that name anymore!)? Your current affairs club? Your bottom? What will go around your waist? What won't? How to avoid throwing up at diaper time? And so it goes with a million other questions seeking priority or at least their own level of importance in your world. But not to worry. Here's the solution:

○ First things first. Establish the order of priority. *You* come first. Without you, nothing works. Attend, then, to your own well-being, appearance, and self-esteem. Get rest when you can, eat properly, and groom yourself daily. Let some other things go, or some other people.

○ Keep your relationship with your co-impregnator alive. Hopefully, it will be a lasting relationship and it will come before any other except that with yourself. Thus, when your baby is grown and gone you will have your mate to cherish instead of a photo album and some baby beads.

○ Love and bond with your baby, but don't make it the focal point of your life. Keep other relationships intact and ongoing and get out into the world in which you are living as soon as possible. Your baby can manage quite well without you while you foray around for a short while. Cabin fever is a deadly bore and satisfies neither mother nor child.

° Avoid help. Now, that is conditional. Sometimes help is really helpful, but often it is not and is oppressive and nerve-racking. It usually depends upon who is supposed to be help-ing. Anyway, too much help for too long is a hindrance. Be prepared in advance to set time limits on help so that you can get it behind you. You are aware, I am sure, of what type of help I am referring to. It is all very personal but can be disas-trous.

° Keep the drawbridge up. Visiting friends and relatives have a way of losing sight of their own experiences, like guests who don't know when to leave at night. Tell tardy friends your doctor insists on extra rest for you. Or tell them you think you have typhoid fever—anything to preserve your privacy when you want it and need it.

° Even if you have had a section, you can usually start some kind of exercise as soon as you get home. Clear it with your doctor and get started as soon as you are allowed to. You can certainly go outside and can attack stairs carefully at any time. So, get outside—weather permitting—as much as you can.

° Unless you have had a section, you can start driving almost anytime your bottom is comfortable enough. Because of the abdominal incision left behind by the cesarian opera-tion, you should avoid driving, even avoid being in the car until your incision has firmed up to the satisfaction of your obstetrician. Sudden stops or starts may damage your stitch-work. Always buckle yourself and your baby in regardless of the local laws. A head-on collision between two cars, each moving at just ten miles an hour, would momentarily increase the weight of an average newborn child to *150 pounds!* Do you think you could restrain that mass?

° As you recall from your hospital experience, your per-sonal hygiene is only slightly restricted. At home, tubs (in-stead of sitz baths), showering, and shampooing go on as always. If you do not enjoy the tub, be sure that your shower includes careful cleansing of the episiotomy area. Avoid communal tubs for a while. You can swim as soon as you are allowed to use a tampon or as soon as your vaginal discharges (lochia) have sufficiently abated. Incidentally, your lochia gradually becomes less bloody and after a few weeks consists mainly of a yellowish discharge. You cannot douche until after your first postpartum visit. If you are not nursing, your first period usually begins four to six weeks after delivery but there are wide variations. Nursing, of course, usually delays the onset of menses by many months.

○ Sex. Before too much time goes by, the call to arms is heard once again around your household. Now, either party in the relationship may issue the first challenge—it varies. No matter. What is to be done about this primal urge and this invitation to skirmish? Well, all the books and instructions that you have seen (and that I have seen) say no sex until after the first postpartum exam, usually some four to six weeks after delivery and therefore about three to five weeks after the first sensual call is heard.

It has been my experience that very few couples wait for official clearance at a postpartum exam before they engage in lovemaking. This is just an observation and should not be interpreted as official clearance or a go-ahead signal. By and large, though, lovemaking is usually safe a few weeks following vaginal delivery without episiotomy, after a few more weeks if an episiotomy has been sustained provided healing is satisfactory, and within a month following a cesarian section. Your obstetrician may have other ideas and you should listen to them no matter what your plans. Remember always, pregnancy is lurking just around the corner—or under the sheets.

○ Continue your regular vitamin/mineral supplement while you are nursing. Take no other medication without your doctor's advice. If your baby is bottle-fed, you should still take a standard vitamin/mineral supplement daily.

○ Work. It has been a general rule that mothers may—or may have to—return to work about six weeks following delivery. This rule is flexible, depending upon the type of work involved, any delivery complications that may have occurred, or any newborn problems requiring special attention.

Such a short time allotted to be spent at home with your baby is a limitation found in the United States alone. All other developed nations provide a much longer maternity leave— some up to a year—with no loss of benefits, seniority, or pension rights at the work place, as stated earlier. Legislation is now before our Congress to change all this and it has an excellent chance of becoming law. Even without legislation, mature organizations are expanding maternity leave benefits and time very rapidly.

When you do have to return to work at whatever time and for whatever reason, your relationship and bonding with your baby does not have to suffer. It is reasonably well established by many studies that what really counts is the amount of quality time you are able to spend with your new responsibility. And that brings up another subject—your time.

At this point in your life, time has become a most precious commodity and must be divided up somehow between competing needs. Unlike the federal budget, there is no provision for deficit time. You have so much of it, you use it or not, and it is gone. Right now you may be rationing it out to a number of roles. You are playing partner, mother, worker, housekeeper, lover, cook, and more—and not necessarily in that order. If your working hours are not flexible, then the others must be. What you have to do is establish their order of importance in your life and allot them your good time as best you can. And ask your partner to share the wealth—and the garbage, the diapers, the supermarket as well as the bed. If you are living alone, you have a few less roles to play but must play them more intensely. Get your priorities right. Give your child all you can give but keep your own life going. You will need it later on. You'll see.

## BONDING

Bonding is a name recently given for an event that always existed between mother and child. Since a title has been awarded to the phenomenon, however, it is necessary that we make some sort of positive statement about it.

Bonding begins between mother and child when the first period is missed, or when the first throw-up occurs, or when the first pregnancy test is positive, or when the fetal heart is seen beating on ultrasound, or heard beating with a Doppler stethoscope, or when the first fluttering movements are detected—somewhere, early on, the *bond* begins.

As pregnancy advances, baby hears and becomes accustomed to its mother's voice and hears and becomes accustomed to the sound of her blood pulsing by the uterus and she becomes accustomed to its movements within her. Thus, at birth they already know each other and have started the bonding process. Likewise, father may feel his baby moving within its mother's abdomen and his baby will learn to recognize his voice as well.

At delivery, if everything is normal and uneventful, the newborn is gently handed to its parents so that they may all see and touch one another. This is not the beginning of bonding or the end. Bonding is a long-term, natural process of which delivery time is but *one* episode.

Some things are important to note here:

○ There is no emotional magic for the infant in rushing skin contact and cuddling. The child's subsequent behavior is not determined by those early moments in the delivery room. No guilt or apprehension, then, should be felt by parents if, for some important reason, early contact must be forgone. This is important to remember. The bonding process is a continuous one and based upon a series of repeated experiences particularly in the first six months of life.

○ Babies that have to be separated from their mothers because of prematurity or other problems have difficulty and are slow to adapt to the bonding process when they are reunited. They also sleep more fretfully and do not feed as well. Such separations are unavoidable, of course, and even then, mothers are encouraged to come to the intensive care nurseries to be with their child.

○ There is some accumulating evidence that overzealous bonding may result in an overdependent child.

So, the bottom line. Enjoy the touch, the feel, the warmth, the movement, and the sound of your child at birth, but do not fret if it is temporarily denied you for whatever reason. Do not make a structured chore or thing about bonding. Remember, experts have destroyed sex, marriage, eating, working, sleeping, and playing by making up rules and guidelines. Don't let them destroy bonding, one of God's little natural joys.

## POSTPARTUM CHECK

This is not your bill. It is your time to be truly released from your obstetrician's bondage, such as it was. You are asked to make this journey between the fourth and sixth week after delivery depending upon some circumstances. The type of delivery and any significant complications that may have existed would be the main determinants of your return time. You should see about an even earlier appointment if:

o Any heavy abnormal bleeding occurs. Usually the vaginal flow decreases regularly after delivery and is about gone in six weeks' time. If your bleeding picks up suddenly, you should call about it. Your first period may befall you toward the end of the six-week waiting period. If you are certain that is what is going on, fine. Otherwise, check it out.

o Fever develops. Elevated temperature may be due to infections in the breasts, kidneys, uterus, legs (phlebitis), lungs, or anywhere. If a section has been performed, peritonitis may overtake you. These infections are uncommon today, but a fever requires an explanation.

o Increased pain occurs. There will be some pains already as you go home. A number of sensitive areas have been altered and healing takes time. However, increased pain in any of these or new areas should be dealt with.

o Depression becomes a problem. As you are already aware, the postpartum blues are of short duration and not a serious problem. Very rarely, significant depression may start after a few weeks of home life (and not necessarily because of it), and help is needed to overcome and shorten this unpleasant complication. Let me stress, this complication is rare.

 ° If you have to travel any distance or if you need for any reason to return to work early.

Your obstetrician will examine you to make sure healing is complete. This involves examination of your pelvic organs and your episiotomy if you had one, and your abdominal incision if you had a section. If it is time for a breast examination or if you have any nursing problems, your breasts will be checked too. You may also be weighed and have your blood pressure taken.

Laboratory tests include a blood count and a Pap smear if either are indicated. Always keep your Pap smear current, and since you are over thirty-five, keep your breast x-rays (mammograms) current as well, provided you are not nursing.

After the examination and tests, you get to chat with your doctor who will likely release you to do a number of things you are already doing but shouldn't be! And remember, just because we all tacitly understand that these facts of life are going on all around us doesn't imply approval or assent—particularly by your own doctor and by me. Things just seem to happen.

One thing you don't want to happen this instant is another pregnancy. So birth control will obviously come up for discussion—that is, if some of the activity mentioned in the foregoing paragraph has not made birth control too late for any discussion other than a philosophical one.

○○○○○○○○○○○○○ **THINGS TO THINK ABOUT** ○○○○○○○○○○○○○

Laboring and delivering in an upright, squatting, or sitting position was an instinctive practice dating back to the beginning of recorded obstetrical history. You may wonder, then, and rightly so, at what point in time and for what reason was the doral recumbency position (flat on your back in bed) introduced?

According to medical historians, sometime in the seventeenth century King Louis XIV of France made it known that he wished to observe his mistress giving birth. Thus, by royal edict, dorsal recumbency became the way to go. Moreover, as operative delivery procedures and anesthesia became more common, so did the continuation and routine use of supine positions.

Anthropological studies show that women, laboring by themselves, assume a variable number of positions. Modern obstetrics encourages freedom in laboring positions, provided that adequate observations of fetal and maternal well-being can be maintained. And no kings will watch you.

○○○○○○○

A recent article about an episiotomy-free society is somewhat startling. Based on the premise that most of the episiotomies now done are unnecessary, it states that about 1.8 million episiotomies could be avoided each year. The resultant saving of hospital time and expenses—let alone the pain—could amount to as much as $36 million each and every year. The $36 million may be a true figure but I doubt it.

Most obstetricians do not do routine episiotomies or routine anything. Such incisions came into practice after hard lessons learned from observing damaging spontaneous tears into the rectum and bladder, and were done in order to spare women from the tragic consequences of such tears. None of us gets paid extra for an episiotomy. It may be more uncomfortable when healing, but the end results justify the vast majority of such procedures. One needs to have watched it both ways for a long time in order to pass judgment. I have.

○○○○○○○

In obstetrics there is a long-standing tradition that all babies must have an Apgar score at one and five minutes after birth. The fetal parameters that are evaluated in obtaining such a score are shown in the accompanying table.

Developed by a very famous pediatrician, the late Virginia Apgar, the scoring technique has served us admirably in the past in assessing the well-being of a newborn infant. However, it is growing out-of-date and Dr. Apgar, just before her death, stated that she felt it was an outmoded tradition that should be replaced by other, more accurate measurements of fetal state. The most likely replacement? Fetal blood gases and Ph determined at birth from umbilical blood samples.

## APGAR EVALUATION METHOD

| Sign | 0 | 4–8 | 10 |
|---|---|---|---|
| Heart rate | absent | less than 100/min | more than 100/min |
| Respiratory effort | absent | weak cry hypoventilation | good strong cry |
| Muscle tone | limp | some flexion of extremities | well-flexed |
| Reflex irritability (response of skin stimulation of feet) | no response | some motion | cry |
| Color | blue/pale | body pink extremities blue | completely pink |

ooooooo

Here is a partial list of the American hospitals recording the largest number of babies delivered in 1985, the last year for which figures are available:

### HOSPITALS WITH OVER 7,000 DELIVERIES DURING 1985

| HOSPITAL | NO. OF DELIVERIES |
|---|---|
| 1. Los Angeles County-University of Southern California, Los Angeles | 17,213 |
| 2. Harris County Hospital District, Houston | 15,736 |
| 3. Parkland Memorial Hospital, Dallas | 12,572 |
| 4. Jackson Memorial Hospital, Miami | 11,678 |
| 5. Magee-Womens Hospital, Pittsburgh | 10,034 |
| 6. Brigham and Women's Hospital, Boston | 9,302 |
| 7. Women and Infants Hospital of Rhode Island, Providence | 7,609 |
| 8. Woman's Hospital, Baton Rouge | 7,562 |
| 9. University of Tennessee Medical Center, Memphis | 7,317 |
| 10. Bexar County Hospital District, San Antonio | 7,099 |

Source: American College of Obstetricians and Gynecologists, "California Hospital Leads in Number of Births, Averages Nearly 50 a Day," *ACOG Newsletter* 31(2):11, 1987.

oooooooooooooooooooooooooooooooooooooooooooooo

# PART 11

# FERTILITY IN THE MIDDLE YEARS

○ 𝕓 ○

# The Question of Fertility

## FERTILITY IN THE FORTIES: FADING FAST

No doubt about it, this time of life complicates the business at hand—childbearing—but more often than not, fortified with wisdom and knowledge, it is an ally. Leaving aside the grace to be found in your maturity, a primelife reproductive experience may be the last rose of all, so it is doubly important to understand the equipment to be traveled with, just how dependable it is, and how likely it is to get everyone there. Further, there is need to know what problems can happen along the way. So, it is necessary to take a straightforward look at the equipment and the potential problems, problems which generally separate into those of conceiving and those of carrying.

First, to the conceiving. Involuntary childlessness increases with age. Although there is no disputing that fact, reliable estimates of the rates at specific age levels are hard to come by. Most collected statistics on the subject are largely historical by the time they see print. Further, the prevalence and voluntary use of reliable contraceptive methods inflates the perceived level of involuntary fertility. The most recent evidence, however, indicates that the following figures are reliable:

| AGE | INFERTILITY |
|-----|-------------|
| 25–29 | 5.5% |
| 30–34 | 9.4% |
| 35–39 | 19.7% |
| 40– | 50.0% |

Although these statistics are as accurate as any obtainable today, they probably do not reflect the rates that actually do now exist. Rapidly increasing medical understanding and technology has certainly increased fertility at all age levels.

## CHANGING PHYSIOLOGY

As the sexual glands (ovaries and testicles) move into the golden years, regressive changes take place which reduce the *total* number of eggs and/or sperm available to form a viable embryo. Not only that, there is a further and regular dilution of germ cell health and vigor so that any union which takes place has less chance of producing a viable embryo. Here are some of the changes:

○ Depletion of mature eggs. Each ovary contains within its substance at the beginning of a reproductive career several hundred thousand eggs. As time goes by, some 400 or 500 of them will, month after month—unless some suppression takes place such as with birth control pills—produce a mature follicle which as it ripens migrates to the ovarian surface and there ruptures into the abdominal cavity looking for a tube to enter. This is, as already delineated, ovulation. It is now clear, however, that only these several hundred specific eggs (germ cells) are capable of maturing and therefore of ovulating. The remaining eggs continue to be more or less immature and although they function in a supportive way and produce certain important ovarian hormones, they can never ovulate. It is clear, then, that when there are no longer any eggs capable of maturation (again, influenced by the pituitary gland) ovulation ceases and under ordinary circumstances sterility becomes absolute. The pituitary gland continues to emit its follicular stimulating hormone (FSH), indeed in ever-increasing amounts. But ovulation does not follow. The store of receptive eggs is gone.

Complete ovarian depletion generally occurs in the late forties (menopause) but it may take place earlier, sometimes many years earlier. Moreover, as shall be seen, there are occasions during menstrual life when ovulation suddenly stops even with plenty of "good" eggs left, only to return quite spontaneously at a later time.

"Wait now," some clever reader is surely saying, "supposing someone takes birth control pills for fifteen years and therefore doesn't ovulate any of those maturable, glorious eggs. What happens when the birth control pills are stopped? Aren't those eggs still there? Can they not go on ovulating for years—even into the sixties and seventies?" No. Not any more than an arm can be preserved for old age by putting it into a cast for twenty years or than a man can save his sperm for old age by avoiding sex in his youth. Not that he would. But he can't.

○ Cessation of spontaneous ovulation. A number of circumstances can prevent spontaneous ovulation even though the ovaries still contain many eggs which are capable of maturing and escaping. Spontaneous ovulation can be suppressed by a number of medicines (e.g., birth control pills), by systemic illnesses (e.g., diabetes), or stressful situations (e.g., jogging). This particular type of suppression is, however, considered pathological and not a physiological process since it is dependent upon and relates to another abnormal condition. But even in the absence of stress, disease, and drugs, spontaneous ovulation will sometimes, without evidence of cause, cease for variable periods of time. Most often, it will reestablish itself just as spontaneously, but as aging progresses, such recovery becomes a less and less likely happenstance.

○ Failed capacity of germ cells to develop. Again, as time multiplies, germ cell viability and vigor does not, and the remaining follicles capable of maturity become less hardy and indeed many may not reach full ripeness and will fail to ovulate. If in fact they do ovulate, they will not fertilize because of diminished vigor within the cell system itself.

○ Genetic defects. The increased stickiness of a chromosome in older germ cells—both ova and sperm—is very well documented and one result, for example, is the most commonly recognized congenital abnormality of all, Down's syndrome. Many other rickety splits in the maturing egg's chromosomal separation system result in genetic abnormalities which are totally incompatible with life and indeed, in many instances, even with fertilization. Such damaged germ cells may be fertilized, die, and be expelled without so much as an abnormal period, let alone signs or symptoms of pregnancy. (See Genetics, pages 249–50.)

○ Changes within the sperm. Each sperm consists of a sperm head which holds nothing much more than concentrated chromosomal tissue and of a tail which propels that tissue to its destiny wherever it may lie. Again, as the vicissitudes of time and whatever take their toll on the testicle and therefore on sperm, not only is the total sperm count reduced, but equally—or more importantly—is their ability to fertilize because of reduced sperm head chromosomal vitality and health. In this regard, then, a *total* sperm count may not be of real value since it may only reflect a *normal* count of an *abnormal* sperm population. The appearance, mobility, and function of the sperm will be of considerably more importance.

○ Reduced sexual exposure. Einstein in his exquisite wisdom once said that any thought, deed, or action could be reduced simply and quickly to a mathematical equation. He may not have had sex in mind at that time or he may have been thinking of it specifically. No matter. The following data, in a rather galling and simplistic way, reveals that sex as a communicative verb can be equated just the way he said. It is clearly seen that physiologically, alas, sexual interplay and therefore sexual exposure and fertility regularly and inexorably, as the distant drummer calls, decline at a rate pleasing to no one.

This considerable physiological event has been alluded to in the past, but because of its sensitive nature, never closely documented. Since society has lifted its prurient lid, however, people have been begging to tell all they can about sex and any other related events, so there is now ample evidence indicating the sexual path and preferences of both men and women. Not all of it concerns us here.

Women generally state that their sexual arousal and enjoyment seems to peak in their thirties and thereafter falls away gradually as menopause approaches. At that time, if exogenous external hormone replenishment is not provided, sexual drive, pleasure, and therefore exposure declines rather abruptly.

Males, on the other hand, exhibit a peak in sexual drive in their twenties, falling away—to coin a phrase—thereafter in a gradual but regular decline as they tumble along reluctantly dragged by a continuing and steady drop of circulating blood testosterone.

Yes, there are wide variations in sexual drive in both sexes and at all ages and generalization always leaves someone out, but not many. The pattern that has been described here is the usual and expected one and well-documented exposure rates now exist for various age levels during a lifetime.

## PATHOLOGY OF INFERTILITY

There are a wide variety of infections and acquired disorders that may ransom reproduction at any stage of the fertile life, some more frequently in youngsters and some as time goes by.

## INFECTIOUS INFERTILITY

The most common pelvic infections that now appear to interfere with fertility are sexually acquired, that is to say, venereal diseases, now commonly called the sexually transmitted diseases (STD). This spectrum of illnesses is so vast that several chapters might be required just to detail the categories and characteristics of each of the prevalent types, a task not possible here. In the past, syphilis and gonorrhea were indeed the major recognizable STD culprits. Syphilis, although again increasing in incidence, has largely been brought under control and is in no way the gruesome destroyer and killer of multitudes that it once was. Not so for gonorrhea. This little bug still constitutes a major public health problem and is surpassed in occurrence rate by few if *any* other infectious diseases. Gonorrhea produces infertility in women by destroying tubal and ovarian architecture, sometimes tragically ending in their complete destruction. Frequently, male infertility follows gonorrhea damage to the prostate gland and to associated structures.

Most gonorrhea responds to appropriate antibiotic therapy, but a new strain introduced into this country from Vietnam is more or less resistant to standard antibiotic therapy. And it is certain that there will be more new strains.

Cytomegalovirus (CMV) is a poorly understood venereal organism which is very difficult to culture and study. It resides in both the male and female reproductive tract and is transmitted solely by sexual intercourse. It produces very few symptoms in either sex—local discharge and irritation mainly—none of which have been thought to have been serious until recently. Now, however, CMV appears closely linked with infertility as well as repeated abortions and fetal wastage, all by mechanisms as yet unclear.

Because of its stubborn cultural characteristics in the laboratory and its extreme difficulty to diagnose, treatment of CMV is difficult and the cure inconclusive. Then how do doctors know it's out there? They know by screening thoroughly a sample population cohort and extrapolating the data thus acquired into large populations—like counting rats in a single row house and multiplying by the number of houses or like gauging a tornado by measuring its swath.

Another complex virus, HTLV III, is involved in the very alarming spread of Acquired Immune Deficiency Syndrome (AIDS). AIDS is today probably the leading medical item in the media—and perhaps rightly so. The ramifications and implications of this disorder, which until recently was found only in homosexuals, Haitians, IV drug users, and some hemophiliacs, are frightening. As an example, the *death* rate from AIDS-associated diseases is greater than that of the ancient and formidable plague! And a mother can give AIDS to her unborn child.

Some mention must be made of herpes. Herpes virus II, which

is known by name to more people in the United States than is their president, has no known *direct* effect upon fertility. It may, however, do some important things to pregnancies as will be seen later on. Herpes virus II is the most common sexually transmitted disease and indeed is probably now the most common infectious disease in the United States—that is, unless it has been replaced by chlamydia.

This inflammation, caused by the sexually transmitted bacteria *Chlamydia trachomatis* and known clinically as NGU (nongonoccocal urethritis), may soon be more common than herpes. Causing few symptoms in male carriers, it usually produces a mildly irritating vaginal discharge in women. It can, however, ascend into the uterus, tubes, and ovaries, and wipe them out. Recently, the diagnosis has been helped by new laboratory tests and the disease fortunately responds to appropriate antibiotics.

There are a number of pelvic and systemic infections of a nonvenereal nature, which can seriously interfere with fertility in both men and women. Toxoplasmosis, for instance, is an infection which is spread in this country generally from infected cat droppings and in Europe and other countries by incompletely cooked meats, particularly pork. The symptoms of toxoplasmosis are those of any systemic viral infection such as influenza or mononucleosis and usually are not in themselves worrisome since they are virtually never fatal or disabling. But toxoplasmosis can have profound effects upon the reproductive systems, both in fostering infertility and fetal damage if a pregnancy exists. The condition is easy to test for (a blood sample) but there is no known treatment—it just runs its course and is gone.

Postabortal infections are becoming significantly less common in this country since the legalization of abortion and the resultant decline of treacherous criminal abortion procedures. Infections, however, still do occur after abortions, particularly those that happen spontaneously and early and go untreated. Such infections may appear minor at the time, but are sufficient to seal off the fallopian tubes and thus block fertilization. Microsurgical correction is sometimes possible after this type of infection.

In a somewhat similar manner to postabortal infections, an intrauterine contraceptive device (IUD) can gradually seal off tubes by stimulating minor, almost unnoticed infections. Many times, this tubal occlusion is not identified until some time after the IUD has been removed. Such an infection, often amenable to surgical correction, is not frequently associated with the IUD. But it happens. At this writing, all IUDs are about to be withdrawn from the marketplace.

There are other more rare forms of pelvic infections which can, by destroying the architecture of the tubes and ovaries, produce infertility. One example of this may suffice and will demonstrate the changing nature of public health and medicine in our country. Tuberculosis of the female pelvic organs used to be a fairly common disorder and a common cause of infertility as well as a tragic chronic disability. Once *un*pasteurized milk disappeared in the United States, thanks to federal regulations, so did almost all pelvic tuberculosis. The availability of tuberculosis-infected milk was surely the cause of this pelvic disease, the bacteria migrating from intestinal involvement of the unfortunate young women afflicted. Government intervention in private affairs is not *always* bad—something worth remembering.

## NONINFECTIOUS INFERTILITY

### Diseases of the ovary

o Endometriosis. This disorder is often present in prime-life, and begins with the formation of little blood cysts in and around the uterus, tubes, and ovaries. The cause still escapes us, but the cells involved in such cysts are like those that normally line the uterus. Whatever the cause, it is a prevalent and painful disorder producing discomfort during the periods, at intercourse, and eventually at other times. It is also coexistent with infertility, even in the early stages, so that its presence probably indicates some accompanying basic factor that produces both endometriosis and infertility. The treatment is either by hormone suppression or by conservative surgery, as long as reproduction remains a goal.

o Other ovarian cysts. There are many other types of ovarian cysts, not all of which interfere with fertility. The polycystic ovary syndrome does. It involves enlarged ovaries covered with a thick capsule which prevents ovulation from taking place. It does, therefore, have a marked effect on fertility. This particular disorder is discovered at laparoscopy examination and is managed either by fertility medications or surgical procedures to the ovaries.

○ Prior surgery to one or both ovaries can influence fertility as well. The surgery may have been for cysts or other destructive disorders. The resultant adhesion formation may interfere with ovulation and interfere with ovum transport through the tube.

## Diseases of the tube

○ Infection. Many of the sexually transmitted diseases today can infect the tubes and close them. This has already been described. Further, it is known that IUDs, even the modern copper IUDs, can produce a silent type of tubal infection which can close the tubes completely. Even if tubal function remains after these and other infections, the jeopardy of an ectopic pregnancy is increased, and that, of course, in turn effects future fertility even more. The older one is in reproductive life, the more likely it is that there has been a previous sexually transmitted disease that could have affected the tubes. It is for just this type of infection that test-tube fertilization techniques have been developed, first overseas and now here.

## Diseases of the uterus

Although not strictly a uterine disease, congenital anomalies or deformities of this organ can interfere with conceiving, conception, and carrying a pregnancy. The uterus forms originally from a midline fusion of two separate reproductive tubes during embryonic organ development. Sometimes the fusion is incomplete and results in a split or double uterus, even half of a uterus (from a single tube). Some of these commonly occurring anomalies can be corrected surgically, some cannot. Of course, these anomalies are not age-related in any way save that they have been present from the very beginning.

More commonly in primelife the uterus may be irregularly studded with fibroid tumors. Fibroids (myomas, myomatas) are benign uterine muscle growths of unknown cause and are present, sooner or later (generally later), in every twentieth white woman and every tenth black. Depending upon their location in the uterine muscle, fibroids can prevent implantation, produce an early abortion, or cause significant vascular problems in late pregnancy. Under correct circumstances, fibroids can be removed (myomectomy) and the uterus spared for future pregnancies.

Sometimes the uterine lining (endometrium) is beset with a single or a vast number of polyps, which are grapelike growths causing irregularities of the uterine lining and generally accompanied by irregular and heavy menstrual bleeding. Such polyps can be simply removed by dilation and curettage (D & C), an outpatient surgical procedure. Sometimes, however, they remain elusive and hard to find.

Previous surgery to the uterus can also interfere significantly with fertility. Fibroid removal, described above, although removing potentially destructive growths, sometimes reduces the uterine cavity or makes it sufficiently irregular that pregnancies have difficulty imbedding, or if this is accomplished satisfactorily, may cause early delivery because of decreased uterine space.

Another not uncommon problem is damage to the lining of the uterus by repeated D & C operations for whatever reason or reasons (polyps, abortions, abnormal bleeding, etc.). The lining (endometrium) is very sturdy and usually regrows without difficulty after repeated insults from a variety of sources including IUDs, oral contraceptives, D & Cs, and infections. However, very aggressive curettage can and does scar the cavity sufficiently to make pregnancy impossible without certain specific treatment. However, it must be pointed out that such operations, while potentially destructive, may be—and often are—lifesaving.

Conization procedures to the cervix (neck of the uterus) in order to control the ever-increasing incidence of precancerous cervical lesions often destroy the integrity of cervical muscle control and pregnancies will drop out through this incompetent cervix long before term. Other surgery already alluded to is, of course, the repair of congenital anomalies and malformations. Previous therapeutic abortions can have two effects on fertility. One is scarring of the endometrium as noted above, and the other is weakening of the cervical canal from repeated dilation, producing the same muscular weakness as conization procedures.

# OTHER GENERAL CONDITIONS AFFECTING FERTILITY

The widespread use of oral contraceptives, as already noted, produced a marked effect upon the reproductive patterns of our society. There have always been questions concerning long-term effects of oral contraceptive therapy upon fertility. It is reasonably well known that prolonged oral contraceptive use (over two consecutive years) may delay the onset of spontaneous ovulation after the pill is discontinued. Further, as use time increases, so does lag time and women who ovulated irregularly before the beginning of oral contraceptive therapy may demonstrate an even greater lag time. No evidence exists that ovulation will not eventually return to most women, but a long time lag is the last thing a primelife candidate needs. The years available for reproduction are regularly slipping away as are all other favorable factors.

## Systemic illnesses

Diseases affecting the general health and well-being of the maternal host are most likely to be present at this time and most of them exert an effect upon pregnancy and, conversely, pregnancy on them. Diabetes, hypertension, cardiovascular renal disorders, and so on all reduce fertility and decreases chances of a healthy pregnancy outcome. These will be dealt with at the proper time farther along. Medications required for the control of systemic disorders also take their toll not only upon fertility and libido, but on the health and well-being of any pregnancy.

## Radiation—chemotherapy

Chemotherapy or radiation for neoplastic disease has very marked and specific effects on the fertility of both sexes. Here are some points:

> o There is no documented increase in congenital anomalies, spontaneous abortion, or pregnancy complications in patients who reproduce after radiation or chemotherapy treatments. Many times, reproductive function returns completely after chemical and x-ray treatment.

○ Large doses of radiation (over 800 rads) always produces permanent sterility. Smaller doses may be followed by recovery.

○ Certain chemicals are more likely to produce sterility than others.

○ Efforts are under way to develop protective isolation of the gonads when radiation or chemotherapy is necessary to control a malignant body process.

○ For more detailed information, consult: *Fertility and Sterility,* Volume 45, April 1986.

## Habits

The use of tobacco, alcohol, drugs, crash dieting, and excessive exercising all have a marked effect upon fertility as well as pregnancy, none of which are good. These too will be dealt with in detail.

## THE BOTTOM LINE

Faced with the formidable array of sterility factors that we have just listed, you might think pregnancy is clearly a state difficult to achieve after thirty-five. True, it is not as easy as it once was. Little is. But there are hundreds of thousands of women who achieve a primelife pregnancy each year in our country and each year their ranks increase. So it is being regularly and successfully accomplished.

All the bad news cast aside, readers are surely more anxious now to know what can be done about infertility problems affecting late reproducers. And in actual fact much help is available.

Infertility study at this time is conducted as it is at any age, except with more haste, and with more study. Because male fertility is somewhat easier to establish, and cheaper to obtain, a sperm count is the first approach. A normal sperm count (60–200 million per cc) with normal mobility (above 70 percent), few abnormal sperm (15 percent or less), and a good volume free of any pus cells points toward a healthy male reproductive system. Sperm transport and hostility studies are done later when indicated (see below). Should the sperm analysis reveal serious defects, female partner studies may be delayed until more evidence of male fertility—or infertility—is developed.

Basic testing of female fertility is directed toward obtaining evidence of both ovulation and tubal patency (opening).

First, ovulation. Absolute evidence of ovulation may be obtained in the office in two ways:

○ An endometrial biopsy taken just before menstruation. This is a common office procedure in which a sample of uterine lining is taken and sent to a pathologist who can determine for certain whether ovulation has or has not occurred. He can also tell how well the endometrium has prepared itself for any oncoming pregnancy. This is a very useful test.

○ A blood progesterone test. Only after ovulation does the ovary make progesterone, some of which gets into the blood stream, in increasing amounts as menstruation approaches. Thus a blood test taken just before menstruation will reveal the presence or absence of progesterone and, therefore, ovulation.

Tubal patency may also be determined in the office in two ways:

○ By a device that can gently push air or $CO_2$ gas through the uterus and, therefore, the tubes under very controlled pressure. Such vapors bubble as they escape the tubes (when they are open) and enter the abdominal cavity. The bubbling is easily heard through a stethoscope on the abdominal wall. Many times the procedure, if positive, is followed in a few moments by shoulder pain as the vapors bubble up under the diaphragm. This is a good secondary sign of patency. If the tubes are obstructed anywhere, no bubbling is heard under any safe pressure and the procedure is abandoned.

○ The same device can be used to pump an oil opaque to x-rays through the uterus and tubes. If the x-ray test is positive, the oil will be seen spilling out into the abdominal cavity. Two advantages of this test are that the site of any obstruction, should one exist, can be identified in either or both tubes and that the cavity of the uterus is outlined so any defect there is visualized.

## WHEN THE BASICS ARE NOT NORMAL

If the repeated sperm count obtained under ideal circumstances (after several days of abstinence and procured in a special condom without lubricants and transported to the lab in warmth within an hour) is significantly abnormal, it will then be necessary to consult either a fertility-oriented urologist or an endocrinologist in order to pursue the problem further.

Commonly, low sperm counts may result from stress, fatigue, tobacco, alcohol and drugs, obesity, or other societal problems. Earlier injuries and infections (mumps, for instance) can have a profound effect upon sperm production as, of course, can many venereal infections. Structural anomalies in the scrotum also can play a role. Finally, a number of medical disorders such as diabetes, anemia, and chronic obstructive lung diseases can interfere significantly with sperm production.

Many of these disorders can be controlled, resulting in a rise in the sperm count, and male fertility returns. Some, unfortunately, cannot.

As with disorders of sperm production, the suppression of ovulation can be laid at many doorsteps. The same societal problems—stress, weight, alcohol, etc.—can supress ovulation. Excessive exercise is particularly damaging to ovulation as is excessive dieting, especially when it leads to anorexia nervosa. Finally, local ovarian disorders, whether infectious, structural, or hormonal, and systemic illnesses will also shut down ovulation.

As in sperm production, many times correction of the overshadowing problem will result in the spontaneous reestablishment of ovulation. Sometimes, however, powerful agents are required to awaken the ovarian tissue. The sophisticated use of drugs has resulted in many successful pregnancies and many multiple pregnancies.

Absence of tubal patency is becoming the most common cause of primelife infertility because of the great increase in pelvic infections related to sexually transmitted diseases. The intense tubal damage done by such infections also makes the tubes most difficult to repair surgically.

Other causes of tubal obstruction are previous surgical procedures on the tubes (ectopic pregnancy surgery or ligation for sterilization, for instance), congenital anatomical defects and, perhaps, the use of IUDs which facilitate the spread of venereal infections.

Modern microsurgical techniques have made it possible to reopen the majority of the tubes that have been surgically closed. The surgery is considerably less successful, however, when infection has been the cause of tubal closure. But in all instances results are constantly improving. When tubal closure cannot be corrected, the modern in vitro fertility clinics may be of help. At these rapidly spreading clinics, eggs are extracted from the ovaries by laparascopic procedures, fertilized in the lab, and inserted into the egg-bearer's uterus to grow and develop. The success rate, while encouraging, is not great.

## IF THE BASICS ARE NORMAL

In the event that the sperm count is normal and both ovulation and tubal patency are proven, we move into an area of more exotic infertility studies. These may include:

o Sperm transport and hostility studies. In this area, fertility specialists look for vaginal and cervical factors that may interfere with the movement of living sperm up into the uterus and tubes. As a further test, sperm is incubated with the female's blood serum to observe for allergic sperm clumping. Positive results in either of these tests require special corrective procedures.

o The use of the hysteroscope and laparascope. A hysteroscope allows easy access to the uterine cavity. It can detect structural abnormalities within that cavity and even allows for correction of many of the defects found. Thus polyps and fibroids within the cavity may be treated with this instrument (which looks exactly like a urologist's cystoscope which, in turn, looks like a large metal soda straw).

o The laparascope, which also resembles a cystoscope, is inserted under anesthesia through the umbilicus and into the abdominal cavity. It allows direct visualization of the whole abdomen and in particular the female pelvic organs. Thus any disorder of the ovaries can be seen as can tubal or uterine disorders. Moreover, inklike dye can be flushed through the tubes (from the uterus) and seen if it spills through the tubes. An obstruction can be viewed and if early endometriosis is present, it too can be visualized, even treated.

° Genetic counseling. Both partners may be submitted to chromosome cultures to determine if genetic abnormalities are contributing to their infertility problem.

This represents only a brief overview of fertility studies employed today to help couples with reproductive problems. Many more-involved procedures and testing are now available but they are beyond the scope of this book.

## SPONTANEOUS ABORTION

Closely related to infertility, of course, is early spontaneous fetal loss or abortion, a common enough accident at any time in reproductive life. It has been held until recently that 20 percent of all pregnancies end in spontaneous abortion. However, an intensive study recently completed indicates that perhaps every other pregnancy aborts. Many of these, of course, happen so early that they produce no symptoms except perhaps a heavy, early period. It required very special study using sophisticated beta HCG and other procedures to arrive at this latest information. So, a spontaneous abortion is unquestionably a common happenstance, and it is also one that increases regularly in frequency as the years go by. Many of the causative factors have been mentioned in the previous sections on infertility but are worth connecting at this time.

### Causes of spontaneous abortion

° *Genetic:* Chromosomes and chromosomal aberrations and abnormalities are found in at least half of the abnormal early abortion embryos. Chromosomal abnormalities may be inborn and always have been present, or may be due to damage of a chromosome from aging, drugs, radiation, delayed fertility, or sporadic chromosomal changes such as nondisjunction and translocation. Such chromosomal abnormalities are scanned fairly efficiently by the human body, and for the most part, aborted spontaneously.

○ *Medical:* Systemic medical illnesses such as diabetes, kidney disease, heart disease, thyroid disorders, and autoimmune response disorders such as subacute lupus erythematosis. All have an increased rate of spontaneous abortion.

○ *The Immune Response:* Pregnancy, remember, is a graft of a foreign embryo on a maternal host. Thus, rejection phenomena are brought about and have to be overcome, and are indeed overcome by a number of suppressive mechanisms which may or may not promptly come into play when required. Certain conditions increase the pregnancy rejection likelihood, and there might be included the presence of abnormal maternal antibodies, ABO blood incompatibilities, antisperm antibodies circulating in the maternal blood, and so on. Many couples plagued with recurrent abortions share significantly more of a certain immune antigen known as HLA. Much work is progressing in this area.

○ *Endocrine Problems:* The most common glandular problem leading to a spontaneous abortion is a progesterone deficiency arising from an inadequate corpus luteum of pregnancy. As you recall, a corpus luteum forms on one ovary at the ovulation site and its duty is to secrete progesterone, the hormone which plays a role in immune suppression mentioned above. Inadequate amounts of progesterone may allow abortion to take place.

Of the other endocrine glands, thyroid disorder, either over- or under-activity, contributes to abortion as well as infertility. These are becoming more rare as thyroid function becomes better understood.

○ *Environmental Factors:* Background radiation and constant exposure to certain toxic substances in the work place and elsewhere increases the abortion rate. Love Canal is a perfect example of the environment and pregnancy. Moreover, certain drugs taken for medical or social reasons induce a higher rate of abortion, particularly in long-term usage.

○ *Infections:* The role of various infections on fertility and abortion has been covered on pages 195–98.

○ *Anatomical.* This area of early fetal wastage has been dealt with on pages 198–200.

° *Miscellaneous.* External or internal trauma or injury of any type, emotional crisis, shock, starvation, exhaustion—all these and many other forces can produce or contribute to abortion.

## Types of spontaneous abortions

° Threatened. There is some light bleeding with cramps, but the cervix is closed and the pregnancy intact.

° Inevitable. The cervix has begun to dilate.

° Incomplete. Some but not all of the products of pregnancy have passed.

° Complete. The uterus is empty and the process complete.

° Missed. There is clear indication of fetal death (usually by ultrasound study), but the uterus fails to empty itself. This situation, untreated, has been known to last from days to years! Not so today.

## Treatment of spontaneous abortion

Only in rare instances where there is a known progesterone deficit is direct treatment indicated in controlling threatened abortion. Usually rest in a quiet environment is all that is suggested. An inevitable or incomplete abortion generally requires a D & C (dilatation and curettage) to remove the dead conception products, reduce blood loss, and reduce the risk of infection. A complete abortion may require no treatment. A D & C is performed by dilating the cervix to a sufficient degree so that the tissues in the uterus may be curetted (scraped away) with safety. Generally, a light anesthetic is given. There is no incision and very little postoperative pain. Most often hospitalization, except as an outpatient, is not necessary. Women who are Rh negative should receive an Rh vaccine after an abortion. (See page 122.) A day or so of rest is required after a D & C and then everything but lovemaking can be resumed.

A missed abortion needs to be removed once the diagnosis is established. This is accomplished by some type of D & C. After an abortion, there is generally a natural and necessary grief response which may involve a guilt component. These feelings are part of the grieving process and should not be suppressed. They are temporary and will pass.

## HABITUAL ABORTION

When a woman experiences three consecutive early fetal losses, there is most clearly a problem of some sort existing, and the designation of habitual abortions is used. The problem may be any one or any combination of the factors that have been listed before. Under these unfortunate circumstances a thorough study and workup by a competent obstetrician or a specialist in infertility problems is indicated. This involves considerable in-depth study, but is important to complete before another pregnancy is attempted. Although the occurrence of three consecutive abortions by chance alone is a possibility, it is not a very great one.

## ECTOPIC PREGNANCY

Remember that when ovulation takes place, the resultant egg must find its way through the abdomen for a short or even long distance into the tube, where it is most usually fertilized and thence on to the uterus to go to bed. Sometimes the trip through the abdomen may involve a considerable journey. For instance, there are cases where women have a tube on one side and an ovary on the other and pregnancy can and does take place under such circumstances. Obviously, the egg has traveled across the lower abdomen to meet its match in the opposite tube.

Although fertilization usually takes place in the tube, it may occur in an ovary or in the abdomen and even when it happens as it should in the tube, the resultant embryo can roll back out into the abdomen for some unknown reason and live there for a while. Finally, and rarest of all, over thirty pregnancies have been reported in women who have previously had their uterus removed! How? Obviously, following the surgery, a microscopic sinus from the back of the vagina into the abdomen must have formed and persisted and thus allowed sperm to migrate to one ovary or another—and bingo! Abdominal or ovarian pregnancies are very rare and, like tubal ectopics, must be interrupted as soon as the diagnosis is confirmed.

So, it is clear perhaps that there are many mechanisms that may produce a living pregnancy outside the uterus, but far and away, the most common ectopic pregnancy resides in one tube or another and is far more likely to be found in the primelife environment than in younger mothers. This is because venereal infection is the leading causative factor of ectopics, and the longer life goes on, the more likely that such infections will have happened. Indeed, there has been an explosion of ectopic pregnancies in the past ten years with no sign of a decrease, all related to the explosion of sexually transmitted diseases.

As outlined in the first section, the symptoms of an ectopic are those of being pregnant, plus bleeding, usually light, and cramping, usually more severe on one particular side. As the pregnancy grows, it is likely to rupture the host tube and produce a surgical emergency with internal hemorrhage and shock. Thus, immediate intervention is indicated once an ectopic pregnancy is diagnosed. The development of modern ultrasound and beta HCG pregnancy testing has made the early diagnosis of an ectopic pregnancy more certain. Surgical removal of the pregnancy is the accepted treatment at this time. With early diagnosis and modern surgical techniques, the tube may possibly be preserved, but great care must be taken. Experimentally, very early proven ectopics have recently been managed by the short-term use of a certain anticancer drug, which destroys all placental tissues and completely avoids surgery! This may be the wave of the future.

The mortality from ectopic pregnancy has declined over recent years, but it is still a considerable cause of maternal loss. Once an ectopic pregnancy has taken place, another one is somewhat more likely. What is more distressing is the fact that once an ectopic has been sustained, the likelihood of a successful term pregnancy thereafter is greatly decreased.

## THE BIG PICTURE

So it would seem from this hostile, bleak discussion that everything imagined and imaginable is against the primelife conception and pregnancy. But that is not so. It only heightens the challenge and therefore sweetens the pot, so to speak, and makes it all the more worthwhile to try. Remember all the other people who have fought all kinds of odds *successfully*—Truman, Robert Bruce, Churchill and England, the Dionne quintuplets, Dr. Defoe, the American Olympic hockey team, Seabiscuit, Frank Sinatra, George Burns, that Oakland kicker, Eleanor Roosevelt, Thomas ("we know 2,000 things that won't work") Edison, Columbus, Gandhi, Beethoven, Milton, Patricia Neal, etc., etc.—and take heart!

○○○○○○○○○○○○○ **THINGS TO THINK ABOUT** ○○○○○○○○○○○○○

Physical forces can alter fertility and pregnancy. For example:

○ High altitudes decrease fertility and produce smaller babies with greater perinatal risk.

○ Electric and magnetic fields, gravity, and acceleration apparently do not adversely interfere with pregnancy.

○ Hyperthermia decreases fertility in males and hot tubs may have harmful effects on the fetus (see page 53).

○ Ionizing radiation (x-rays, etc.) can, of course, have disastrous effects on fertility and pregnancy.

○ Noise has no known effect on pregnancy nor does its high-level companion, ultrasound, thank goodness.

○ Optical and microwave radiation (ultraviolet, infrared, lasers, video display terminals [VDTs], and microwave ovens) does not penetrate deeply enough to damage a fetus in any way. There has been a recent stir about VDTs and clusters of obstetrical problems related to them, but no reliable evidence yet exists one way or the other.

○ Vibration. Don't put away your vibrators. Studies of the worst vibrations of all—truck driving—failed to correlate with any reproductive damages. No one has yet studied the effects of hard rock music—no one can get close enough!

○ Physical abuse. Over 10 percent of the pregnant women at one eastern maternity clinic reported physical abuse in their relationship. Of these, 21 percent reported increased abuse during pregnancy, 36 percent reported less. Injuries were about the face (99 percent), arms, legs, abdomen, breasts, and back. They included bruises, lacerations, broken bones, and lost teeth. Pregnancy outcome was not significantly altered in these women. Neither were their partners' faces.

○○○○○○○

A recent study implicates routine vaginal douching (once a week or more) as a causative factor in ectopic pregnancy. The risk was apparently greater with commercial douche preparations.

○○○○○○○

Can men exposed to a variety of chemical and physical agents while at work, at play, or under medical treatment affect the success and health of their future offspring? This is quite possible and seems a reasonable assumption. The sum of recent studies indicates that many of the same hazards which affect women's reproductive health—radiation, mutagenic chemicals, narcotics, and alcohol—can work their biological damage on men's reproductive harvest as well.

○○○○○○○

Flying in commercial aircraft has been accused of causing many potential obstetrical hazards, particularly among stewardesses who theoretically are exposed to greater ozone and ultraviolet showers, less oxygen saturation, drier air, time zone and circadian shifts, turbulence, hard work, and so forth. Little substantial evidence has been accumulated to support these claims and in fact pregnant stewardesses are now allowed to work much later in their pregnancies than in the past. The pregnant airline passenger is probably much safer in a commercial jet than in her own environment.

○○○○○○○

Diseases, like humans, are born and die. Legionnaire's disease and AIDS are two recent births, while smallpox and perhaps poliomyelitis represent two recent deaths. Rubella (German measles) is a common virus that we have the opportunity and obligation to put to death. Although a relatively mild viral infection, it can profoundly damage a fetus *in utero.* In the 1964–65 U.S. epidemic, there were over 11,000 fetal deaths by abortion (spontaneous or therapeutic) and 20,000 infants born with congenital rubella disease, and the epidemic cost us $1.5 billion! The disease can be wiped out by a readily available, safe vaccine contraindicated only during pregnancy or when pregnancy is contemplated within three months.

○ ○ ○ ○ ○ ○ ○

Although all the figures are not in, it is quite likely that there were less than 200 maternal deaths in the United States last year. This is a phenomonally low figure when weighed against the fact that there were 3.6 million deliveries, over 2 million elective abortions, and untold millions of spontaneous abortions! A remarkable statistic.

Some of these maternal deaths were due to anesthetic complications, some to uncontrolled bleeding, some to infection, some were complications of abortions, and some were medical complications. Some were preventable, some were not.

Maternal mortality is declining at a phenomenal rate: It is thirty times less than it was in 1940, and has declined 68 percent in the last ten years. Hospital-based or hospital-supported deliveries account for 99 percent of all maternity care in the United States, and prenatal care is available almost everywhere except the inner core of large metropolitan areas. Anyone wishing to belittle the value of prenatal care and hospital-supported deliveries and to harken back to the good old days might want to ponder the following: There exists now—here in the United States—a religious sect which, for their own reasons, allows their pregnant women *no* prenatal care and *no* trained attendants to deliver them. All of the deliveries are managed at home with just casual help! This is all very true, or I would be in deep trouble just for telling it. At any rate, recent studies show that infant mortality in this religiously managed group is *three times greater,* and that (difficult to believe) maternal mortality is *ninety* times greater than that which exists in the rest of the state that harbors this group! And Arkansas is not the state.

So much for home deliveries. While we are talking, alas, of death, here are some other statistics that might put maternal deaths into some perspective:

○ In the same year that we lost 200 mothers, we lost 5,000 joggers and 1300 bicyclists. Lightning killed 104.

○ Also in that year, toys claimed 31 children's lives and injured 587,000 others.

- Suicide claims 72 victims each day—and is rising.
- Alcoholism killed 276 youngsters between ages 15 and 19 in 1984.
- On Christmas Eve and New Year's Eve, 1984, there were 259 traffic fatalities—half of them alcohol related.
- Five hundred people freeze to death each year.

Reproductive mortality is a more comprehensive way of expressing all female deaths due to the reproductive environment, and it therefore includes maternal deaths, contraceptive deaths, and deaths from sexually transmitted diseases. The most recent figures show pregnancy accounting for 42 percent of the total, contraception 38 percent, and STD 20 percent. The last two groups are constantly increasing, while the first is declining.

And among all these tragic figures only maternal mortality is constantly decreasing.

Finally, it is important to note that maternity mortality risk increases in the primelife—increases significantly. Analysis of these deaths indicate that lack of adequate prenatal care and the presence of complicating systemic diseases are the major sources of this mortality. A healthy, well-cared-for primelife mother should suffer no mortal risk in pregnancy and delivery—at least no more than any mother at any age. And that risk, as you can see, is minimal.

○ ○ ○ ○ ○ ○ ○

Recently, in another country, a pair of fraternal twins were diagnosed—one male and one female. The male was determined by chorionic villi sampling (see pages 252–53) to be at risk for hemophilia. It was selectively aborted by transabdominal techniques and the female twin went to term and delivered normally.

○ ○ ○ ○ ○ ○ ○

Speaking of twins, it may be that many more pregnancies than realized begin as twins. Recent ultrasound studies indicate that possibility, suggesting that one twin or the other may be resorbed without incident at a very early stage of pregnancy.

○ ○ ○ ○ ○ ○ ○ ○ ○ ○ ○ ○ ○ ○ ○ ○ ○ ○ ○ ○ ○ ○ ○ ○ ○ ○ ○ ○ ○ ○ ○ ○ ○ ○ ○ ○ ○ ○ ○ ○ ○ ○ ○ ○ ○

# PART III

# MEDICAL GUIDANCE
# AND MONITORING

# ○ 7 ○

# Medical and Surgical Complications

Primelife mothers are somewhat more likely to have sustained a chronic medical condition by the time they become pregnant. Most of these acquired conditions (although some are congenital—see Heart Disease, pages 229–31) have an effect upon pregnancy just as pregnancy most likely has an effect upon the medical disorder. This section deals with most of the common primelife medical conditions which must be faced during pregnancy.

## DIABETES

Prior to the discovery of insulin in 1922, pregnancy and diabetes could not coexist. Survival was virtually impossible. Diabetes by itself signaled a short and unpleasant life span at best. Insulin changed all that.

The first report of pregnancy associated with insulin-controlled diabetes appeared in 1933. It recorded a maternal mortality of 10 percent and a fetal mortality of 50 percent—not good, but better. Gradually the statistics have improved. Even so, recent textbooks describe pregnancy in diabetics as a circumstance of significant maternal jeopardy associated with decreasing maternal survival accompanied by increasing severity of the diabetes and further accompanied by substantial fetal mortality and morbidity.

Primelife mothers, who are unfortunately more likely to be

diabetic, can take heart. This bleak picture has dramatically changed in the 1980's. Properly controlled and properly complying, the outlook for a pregnant diabetic and her offspring is virtually the same as for her nondiabetic counterpart. The key is to keep blood sugar levels in the normal range at all times—*euglycemia* is the medical term.

Pregnancy itself is normally accompanied by a mild degree of glucose (sugar) intolerance, which increases as pregnancy advances and is due to the development of insulin resistance in all maternal tissues. This fact explains why some mothers may become, at least temporarily, diabetic during late pregnancy. This condition is called *gestational diabetes* and is described shortly. This fact also explains, at least partly, why a diabetic's insulin requirements change and vary throughout pregnancy.

What can inadequately controlled diabetes do to a fetus?

○ Increase the incidence of congenital malformations.

○ Cause abortions and premature deliveries.

○ Produce large babies (macrosomia) and thus difficult deliveries.

○ Increase intrauterine fetal death.

○ Make fetal existence very tenuous and difficult after birth.

And what can inadequately controlled diabetes do to the mother?

○ Markedly increase the risk of acidosis, hyperglycemia (excess blood sugar), and insulin reactions.

○ Advance the course of vascular deterioration in the eyes, kidneys, and the general vascular tree.

○ Increase the risk of obstetrical complications such as hypertension of pregnancy, hydramnios, and obesity.

Good results are dependent upon good management. You will need to cooperate by:

○ Adhering to strict dietary control to prevent excess weight gain, acidosis from starvation, and to help provide normal glucose levels.

° Maintaining insulin dosage arranged in a multiple component plan to again keep glucose levels normal day and night.

° Balancing between food intake, insulin dosage, and physical activity.

° Self-monitoring of glucose levels four to eight times daily.

° Checking out the cause of acidosis carefully.

° Reporting any fever or infection promptly.

° Regular visits (probably weekly) with your obstetrician and/or internist.

Your obstetrician's role:

° Your obstetrician will want to see you very frequently, perhaps weekly. The progress of your pregnancy and the control of your diabetes will be closely monitored. Blood tests for a certain type of hemoglobin will be taken to determine your long-term glucose control. Your blood pressure, kidney function, and visual health will be checked.

° Ultrasound determinations are usually made at the initial visit and regularly thereafter to observe for congenital anomalies or amniotic fluid volume changes. Later ultrasound will determine fetal state by means of the biophysical profile. See pages 259–60.

° Hospitalization may be instituted in the face of very difficult glucose control or if infections or hypertension occurs.

° Tests for fetal well-being in the third trimester will involve not only the biophysical profile, but stress and nonstress testing and perhaps amniocentesis for evidence of fetal lung maturity.

° Labor is usually allowed to take place on its own unless some complication comes along. Evidence of fetal distress, postmaturity, macrosomia, and maternal hypertension would all indicate induction of labor or cesarian section. Most sections, however, are done for purely obstetrical indications.

&#9702; Generally, a pediatrician or neonatologist is present at delivery or soon after to manage the newborn.

These are wide variations in all these management principles and none of them are hard and fast. Nor are they gospel. Nor is your obstetrician remiss, if he/she does less testing or more testing.

## GESTATIONAL DIABETES

You already know that pregnancy is normally accompanied by a mild state of glucose intolerance. In about 3 percent of all pregnant women, this intolerance reaches a point that is considered abnormal. Such women have gestational diabetes (GD). Here are some points to consider:

&#9702; Primelife mothers are more likely to have gestational diabetes.

&#9702; Even though the glucose tolerance may return to normal after delivery, all GDs must be treated during pregnancy as diabetics.

&#9702; More than half of all GDs will sooner or later become true diabetics.

&#9702; All patients with GD are at greater risk for developing fetal macrosomia (large babies).

&#9702; Intrauterine death and newborn mortality are significantly increased in GD.

&#9702; Mounting evidence also indicates that long-term offspring complications include obesity and diabetes.

In view of these significant problems associated with gestational diabetes, it is important that all primelife mothers be screened for abnormal glucose intolerance as follows:

&#9702; Between twenty-four and twenty-eight weeks of pregnancy, blood samples are taken an hour after mother is forced to drink a wretched concoction containing a measured amount of glucose. If the blood sample reveals unusually high levels of glucose, then a full-scale blood glucose tolerance test is ordered. If it reveals abnormally high values, we have GD.

° Other tests are under study which may reveal abnormal glucose intolerance earlier in pregnancy, as early as ten weeks. Such tests are not yet in general use. A glucose tolerance test before twenty-four weeks is, of itself, not reliable.

Gestational diabetes, detected and managed as a diabetic would be managed, is not accompanied by any increase in maternal or fetal complications. Such management includes:

° Nutritional and dietary counseling similar to a diabetic program.

° Prevention of excess weight gain.

° Insulin therapy when diet alone does not control excessive blood glucose levels.

° Proper monitoring of fetal well-being as in diabetics.

° Delivery intervention when indicated.

° Breast-feeding whenever possible.

° Follow-up evaluation of glucose tolerance at regular intervals.

° Counseling about further pregnancies.


## OBESITY

For thirty-years, I have instructed my office staff to completely and forever avoid two words when dealing with our patients. The two words? *Fat* and *old.*

Now, regardless of my instructions, aging (and therefore growing old) has continued on with my patients at the same steady pace. No increase.

Not so, unfortunately, has fat. My patients and indeed all Americans are getting fatter and fatter. Obesity is twice as common as it was thirty years ago! It appears that the health-conscious have become leaner, but everyone else has become fatter. And obesity (defined as weighing 200 plus pounds) has profound effects upon pregnancy.

° Fertility decreases while spontaneous abortion increases.

° Pregnancy detection is difficult as is the observation of normal pregnancy growth and development.

° Medical complications such as hypertension and diabetes are more common.

° Obstetrical complications are immense and include the following:

Preeclampsia (hypertension of pregnancy)
Twins
Macrosomia with difficult delivery
Poor labor
Anesthesia difficulties of all types
Postpartum bleeding
Poor wound healing
Thrombophlebitis
Increased need for cesarian section

There is little that can be done to help obese women through their pregnancies. However, seen before pregnancy, they should be assisted in a vigorous, controlled weight-loss program and advised not to conceive until weight stability has been achieved for several months.

Obese mothers can and do mobilize their own food stores during pregnancy and thus may be encouraged to eat less and to gain only twelve to fifteen pounds throughout pregnancy. This goal is easier to state than achieve or they wouldn't be where they already are. On *no account* should weight loss be attempted while pregnant. No benefits will accrue to either party, particularly the fetus.

## LUNG DISORDERS

Lung physiology undergoes impressive changes during pregnancy. As a result, chest breathing largely replaces abdominal (diaphragmatic) breathing and further, there is a much greater volume of air exchanged each minute as pulmonary resistance decreases. Despite these improvements in air exchange, any acute or chronic airway obstructive disorder during pregnancy produces a marked increase in the breathing workload. Chronic bronchitis, asthma, and emphysema represent the usual chronic obstructive processes while acute bronchitis and pneumonia represent the acute insults. Any lung disorder can have a profound effect on fetal and maternal health and should be treated very diligently and with great respect.

## CHRONIC PULMONARY DISORDERS

### Asthma

Probably 1 percent of primelife mothers are asthmatic and have learned to live with and (as much as possible) control the disorder. Pregnancy has variable effects on asthmatics but most often deterioration is more common than improvement. It is more difficult for the bronchioles to clear themselves and overinflation often occurs. There also appears to be a slightly greater risk of status asthmaticus, a condition where acute respiratory obstruction takes place and heroic efforts are needed to bring it under control. Here are some further points about asthma:

○ Fetal effects are variable, but it is generally noted that there are more abortions, more preterm deliveries, and more small babies for dates.

○ Over 5 percent of the infants born of asthmatic mothers develop asthma.

○ Asthmatics are more likely to develop status asthmaticus when:

Exposed to fresh paint
They ingest aspirin or nonsteroidal anti-inflammatory drugs
They don't follow instructions
The severity of the asthma is underrecognized
An upper respiratory infection occurs
In the presence of allergies, emotional stress, exercise, and lung irritants

○ Cortisone may be necessary to control asthmatic attacks during pregnancy. The amount used has not been associated with significant birth defects. Certainly, uncontrolled asthma has greater fetal and maternal risks than cortisone.

° Asthma during labor can be managed with regular medications given through the intravenous line.

  ° Asthma is not a contraindication to breast feeding, but maternal medications must be given cautiously.

## Emphysema and chronic bronchitis

Most often, these progressive lung disorders are associated with prolonged cigarette smoking. Emphysema results in loss of elasticity of terminal breathing sacs and thus permanently decreases the transfer of air through the lungs. Chronic bronchitis is destructive to the bronchial tubes that transport air to the terminal breathing sacs. In either case, the absorption of oxygen and removal of carbon dioxide becomes increasingly difficult.

Pregnancy does not hasten the progression of either disorder, but babies born to mothers thus afflicted are smaller for dates and may be slower to develop. Both lung disorders are more likely to be found in primelife mothers who have been addicted to nicotine for any substantial time.

## ACUTE PULMONARY DISORDERS

### Influenza

For some unknown reason, pregnant women are more likely to succumb to influenza, and further, the infection is more likely to be severe and long lasting. Influenza is a virus transmitted by nasal secretions and generally works its will in the winter months and only in temperate climates. The three influenza strains, A, B, and C, can appear in different combinations, variations, and locations during any given year and that is how each epidemic is designated. Thus, the notorious swine flu epidemic was caused by the following virus: A/N.J./8/76(Hsw1N1). This indicates that type A virus was involved, that it first appeared in New Jersey (actually in the barracks at Fort Dix), that it was identified in August 1976, and that it had some particular genetic aberrations (Hsw1N1) that required a special vaccine. The rest is history.

Here are some things you should know about the flu.

° The disease usually lasts four or five days and is gone, but may be followed by several weeks of fatigue and weakness, particularly during pregnancy. Also, during pregnancy (and particularly with type A virus involvement) primary influenza pneumonia is more likely to take place. This is a very serious type of pneumonia.

° Routine vaccination of pregnant women is no longer advised. However, should the pregnancy be complicated by chronic lung disorders, diabetes, or cardiovascular disease, vaccination is recommended. Preventive vaccination is also advised in the face of a confirmed oncoming epidemic only when the proper vaccine is available. Last year's vaccine is usually no good for this year's influenza. Modern vaccines, incidentally, are very safe and generally do not produce flu symptoms as the older products did.

° A drug called amantadine prevents or modifies type A influenza and should be considered for pregnant women who are sensitive to egg protein and thus cannot take the vaccine—since it is grown in eggs—or are in the midst of an epidemic and thus will not be protected quickly enough by a vaccine.

° Amantadine has not been proven safe during pregnancy, but for pregnant women in high-risk situations, the benefits would seem to outweigh the risks.

° During influenza epidemics, pregnant women should avoid any public gathering, close contact with anyone, handrails, doorknobs, elevator buttons, and any other surfaces touched by other hands.

## Pneumonia

Once a common and serious disorder, pneumonia has retreated into the wings since the advent of antibiotics. Still, it complicates about 1 pregnancy in 1000 and it can significantly damage mother and baby.

° Pneumonia is poorly tolerated by pregnant women and thus complications with prolonged recovery rates are not unusual.

○ Premature labor is a common complication of pneumonia and takes place when the respiratory strain can be least tolerated.

○ The pneumococcus bacteria has always been and still is the most common bacteria involved in acute pneumonia. Recent evidence, however, implicates the Legionnaire bacteria in up to 20 percent of all recent pneumonias and, indeed, this type of pneumonia is now being reported in pregnancy. Sadly, other types of deadly pneumonias are also being reported in pregnant women who are afflicted with AIDS.

○ Prompt treatment with the appropriate antibiotics brings most maternal pneumonias to a halt, but premature labor must be watched for very carefully.

## RENAL DISEASE

Kidney disorders are very common in pregnancy and prime-life mothers are more likely to have sustained preexisting kidney diseases, which may flare up while they are carrying their child. It is therefore very important that kidney function and health be closely monitored as pregnancy moves along. Here are some changes that pregnancy induces in kidney anatomy and physiology:

○ The kidneys increase in size and remain enlarged throughout pregnancy.

○ The ureters (pencil-sized tubes which conduct urine from the kidneys to the bladder) begin to dilate in early pregnancy and the flow of urine through them is impeded, thus increasing the chance of infection.

○ Kidney filtration doubles in order to handle the excretory needs of both mother and fetus.

### Pyelonephritis

Probably the most common severe kidney complication in pregnancy is pyelonephritis, which is a bacterial infection of one or both kidneys. This disorder is the number one reason for nonobstetric hospital admission during pregnancy.

Pyelonephritis can lead to more profound maternal infection and to fetal damage from maternal fever, the necessary antibiotics, or from premature labor as a result of the infection.

When bacteria are discovered in the urine of primelife mothers by routine testing, vigorous treatment is indicated. The presence of bacteria in the urine, even without symptoms, indicates the potential for spread upward and thus pyelonephritis. So routine urine checks for bacteria are important and can be done in the doctor's office. The symptoms of acute pyelonephritis are chills, fever, and back pain, usually associated with painful and frequent urination. You should report such symptoms promptly.

Appropriate antibiotic therapy generally halts pyelonephritis. Whether such therapy needs to be continued after the infection subsides is a matter best determined by your obstetrician.

Cystitis (bladder infection) is also accompanied by painful and frequent urination, often with blood in the urine. Cystitis, however, is not generally associated with fever or back pain. Although it is not nearly as serious as pyelonephritis, the one can lead to the other, so vigorous and prompt treatment is in order.

If you have been afflicted with previous kidney infections, you are more likely to have reinfections while you are pregnant and will require special observation and testing.

## Chronic pyelonephritis

This disorder, as previously stated, may well involve primelife mothers. Repeated kidney infections can result in the destruction of kidney tissue and therefore forever reduce kidney function. Thus, the strain of pregnancy may not be answerable. Kidney function tests can usually tell in advance whether a successful pregnancy can be maintained and whether it is safe to even contemplate such a step.

## Other renal conditions

There are certain unusual kidney disorders that can affect pregnancy or be affected by pregnancy. Thus, single kidneys, cystic kidneys, and kidneys disordered by diabetes or lupus erythematosis all require special attention by your obstetrician.

Pregnancy associated with kidney grafts were once very rare, but now over 1000 cases have been reported. Usually the pregnancies are successful but there may be significant complications. Most problems are due to immunosuppression, which, of course, is necessary to insure that the kidney graft is not rejected. Most obstetricians counsel no pregnancy for at least one year after a living transplant and two years after a cadaver transplant. Delivery is by cesarian section because the transplanted kidney is snuggled into the pelvis so as to be more safely joined to the bladder. But it all works out.

## HIGH BLOOD PRESSURE

Because of the way life unfolds, primelife mothers are more likely to have sustained permanent insults of one type or another to their cardiovascular systems. The resultant disorders can have a marked effect upon pregnancy just as pregnancy can unfavorably alter the particular disease which has damaged the heart and vascular system. The interplay of one upon the other must be carefully monitored as pregnancy progresses.

### Chronic hypertension

Preexisting high blood pressure from whatever cause can have profound effects on pregnancy outcome.

° Superimposed hypertension of pregnancy is much more likely to take place.

° Intrauterine growth retardation (IUGR) is increased fourfold. (See pages 133–34.)

° Abnormal stress tests are more commonly seen.

° Premature separation of the placenta (abruptio placenta) and intrauterine fetal death are not infrequent complications of chronic hypertension.

Management of this dangerous pregnancy complication includes:

° Appropriate and frequent prenatal visits with assessment of the hypertensive problem and the many medical complications associated with it.

° Medications to control unusually high blood pressure

episodes. Such medications vary and are best managed by your own doctor, in consultation with an appropriate specialist if indicated.

o Frequent blood pressure observations to detect the potential onset of superimposed hypertension of pregnancy.

o Stress and nonstress testing along with ultrasound procedures to detect evidence of fetal distress.

o Early delivery by the safest route if the uterine environment proves too hostile.

o Hypertensive patients who wish to nurse and who require antihypertensive drugs may usually plan on nursing since there are certain blood pressure medications which do not pass readily into breast milk. But such a medication program must be individually tailored and is not always successful.

## HEART DISEASE

One hundred years ago, textbooks of obstetrics rarely mentioned heart disease as a complication of pregnancy. Although plenty of heart disease existed, there were just too many other obstetrical problems to worry about.

Fifty years ago, obstetrical texts were vitally concerned with heart disease and its effects on pregnancy. At that time, *acquired* heart disease was the most common obstetrical cardiac complication, with *congenital* heart disorders running a poor second. Almost all the acquired heart disease was caused by rheumatic fever, which, in turn, was the result of a childhood streptococcus throat infection. Penicillin virtually wiped that disease away and with it most rheumatic heart disease. We rarely see it today.

Congenital heart disease and pregnancy were, as noted, rare complications because there was no treatment to salvage the congenital heart patient. Modern cardiac surgery has drastically altered that picture, and as a result, there are more and more mothers with stabilized congenital heart lesions who are carrying pregnancies. Moreover, the incidence of congenital heart disease is not declining. If anything, it is increasing. And children born of mothers with congenital heart disorders are slightly more likely to sustain congenital heart lesions themselves. Thus, this area of heart disorders during pregnancy is expanding and challenging.

So we come to the present. Primelife mothers with heart disorders are pregnant at a time when vast improvements in cardiology diagnosis and management are in place. Such advances provide the opportunity to carry pregnancy to full term, in most instances with safety to both mother and child. Here is some more information:

° The heart is, of course, vastly affected by pregnancy. It works harder and faster, putting out more blood on each stroke and sustaining a much larger circulating blood volume.

° The most usual mix of heart diseases in primelife is congenital, arteriosclerotic, and rheumatic, the last two being acquired heart disorders and still together accounting for two thirds of all cases. Rheumatic heart disease used to account for 95 percent all by itself. It now constitutes a small portion of acquired heart disease.

° No matter what type of heart disease is present, rest, weight control, avoidance of tobacco, and prevention of anemia and of infections are very important principles to follow.

° Certain medications are often required to manage the heart problem associated with pregnancy. They are given with great care since some of them have serious fetal side effects. One group of them, the oral anticoagulants, must not be used at all.

° There is a greater risk for premature labor, small babies for dates, and slow-to-grow babies. Babies born of congenital heart-diseased mothers, as we have seen, are more likely to have congenital heart disease themselves. A well-compensated cardiac mother can expect the same fetal survival as any primelife mother. However, when the degree of heart disease results in very considerable maternal disability, the fetal survival rate is diminished. A 10 to 30 percent fetal loss is recorded in this risky area. Therapeutic abortion is rarely necessary in the management of pregnant cardiacs today.

° Pregnancy may be undertaken after all kinds of cardiac surgery, even after coronary bypass operations. Further, should it become necessary, open-heart surgery is possible and indeed is done during pregnancy. The maternal risk here is no greater, but depending on the type of heart surgery, the fetal outcome may be in jeopardy.

o Women with mitral valve prolapse should expect to live normal lives. Most primelife mothers with MVP will have uneventful pregnancies and normal deliveries. An antibiotic regime is usually recommended around the time of delivery.

## ANEMIAS

A red blood cell is born in the bone marrow, and when it is mature and filled with hemoglobin, it is pushed out into the general circulation where it carries oxygen to all parts of the body. Several weeks later it expires, the hemoglobin it contained becomes bilirubin (which is yellow and explains why your bruises turn yellow as the red blood cells within them decompose), and the cycle starts all over again.

Reduction in the total body red-cell mass is called anemia and indicates an underlying disorder of some sort. Blood may be produced too slowly (nutritional or bone marrow disorders), destroyed too fast (hemolytic anemia), or be lost to the body by bleeding from some source.

### Nutritional anemias

Iron deficiency is responsible for 95 percent of *all* pregnancy anemias. Women at best live on the verge of iron deficiency. They have a small iron storage capacity and lose a significant amount of it during cyclic bleeding. Pregnancy represents a state of negative iron balance for them which cannot be replaced by nutritional means alone. Thus, iron supplementation is very important. Sometimes oral iron is not enough and sometimes it produces sufficient gastrointestinal and dermatological side effects that women avoid its regular use. Under such circumstances, intramuscular iron must be given. This is a safe though unpleasant way to achieve the iron stores needed for both fetal and maternal needs.

Folic acid deficiency will also produce a significant pregnancy-related anemia. Folic acid is a water-soluble vitamin necessary for normal red blood cell formation, and it is the *most common* vitamin deficiency in our society. About 15 percent of all pregnant women have evidence of folic acid inadequacy. Fortunately, almost all prenatal vitamin/mineral supplements contain the total daily needs of folic acid. Take your pill and don't worry.

## Hemolytic anemia

Sickle cell disease is an inherited chronic hemolytic anemia that is confined almost exclusively to blacks. Not only is anemia present, there are as well recurrent attacks of painful joints and of severe abdominal pain crisis often confused with surgical conditions such as acute appendicitis.

The life expectancy in sickle cell disease has been such that not many survived long enough to be primelife mothers. However, modern care has extended life for these individuals and, indeed, has made pregnancy safer for both mother and child. Meticulous and close care is necessary throughout such a pregnancy.

## Purpura

An occasional primelife pregnancy may be complicated by ideopathic thrombocytopenic purpura (ITP). This is coincidental since the one does not cause the other, but ITP generally affects women of childbearing years, pregnant or not. Normally circulating blood contains tiny cells called platelets without which blood will not clot. ITP is an autoimmune disorder that destroys platelets and, as it does, the coagulability of blood decreases. Thus, spontaneous bruising (purpura) appears and bleeding may occur from a number of body sources. Unchecked, ITP can be fatal. Fortunately, treatment is almost always successful. But there are some pregnancy complications.

Cortisone is often necessary to restore the platelet count to reasonable levels. Fetal effects must be considered. When cortisone is not effective, a splenectomy (removal of the spleen) may have to be resorted to. The spleen, it appears, is largely responsible for the platelet destruction.

Fifty percent of newborn babies also have some temporary signs of ITP. Male circumcision must be delayed and breast feeding should be avoided. Usually the infant's platelet counts are normal within a few weeks.

Although the platelet count normally drops somewhat during pregnancy, and thus bruising is more likely, you should report any unusual shower of spontaneous bruiselike episodes.

## CANCER

Cancer and pregnancy are not unusual companions and, sadly, more likely to be met together in the primelife. Such a combination is a traumatic emotional experience for patient and physician and it demands the closest interdisciplinary approach that medicine has to offer.

Although any cancer can complicate pregnancy, usually it is cervical (2 percent), or breast (1 percent) in origin. It should be noted, though, that 5 to 15 percent of women with Hodgkin's disease will get pregnant some time during the smoldering course of the disease. Malignant melanoma and ovarian cancer constitute the other cancers usually seen in pregnancy. Sadly, before *this decade* is out, lung cancer will supplant *all others* as the most common in pregnancy. This is already true in one state. Some further facts:

○ Regular Pap smears and mammography examinations should be as routine for you as brushing your teeth. Annual Pap smears can prevent invasive cervical cancer. Mammography can safely detect breast lesions at an early stage where control is possible. Routine mammography is at present contraindicated during pregnancy, but that is changing. Moreover, new techniques for early detection of breast disease, which are safe to use in pregnancy, are on the way.

○ The primary purpose of therapy is to destroy the cancer and preserve the fetus. In some stages of neoplastic disease, this represents a difficult challenge and compromises must be made. Thus treatment is sometimes modified (with the mother's consent, of course) to give the unborn babe a few weeks more growing time. In other instances, a baby may be delivered several weeks early in order to get to work on a manageable tumor.

○ Women who have had breast cancer treated and controlled for two or three years may consider a pregnancy, except that primelife mothers should have individual multidisciplinary consultation before embarking upon a pregnancy.

○ Therapeutic abortion or other early termination of pregnancy apparently does not affect the course of breast cancer one way or the other. Mothers treated for breast cancer should not nurse.

○ Quit smoking.

The management of cancer during pregnancy is very involved, and this brief overview can only touch the surface. Mothers facing this combination of conditions should be managed in tertiary care (see pages 240–41) centers whenever possible.

"An ounce of prevention is worth a pound of cure." Nowhere in the world is this trite aphorism more true.


## EPILEPSY

About 1 primelife mother in 100 enters pregnancy with a seizure disorder, almost always epilepsy of one form or another. Epilepsy occurring in pregnancy only (gestational epilepsy) is exceedingly rare and is minor in seizure type.

Here are some more strange things about pregnancy and epilepsy:

○ About half the patients have no increase in seizures while pregnant; 30 to 40 percent have more; the rest, less.

○ Women who suffer from increased seizures during menses are likely to have more attacks during pregnancy.

○ Epileptic mothers carrying male infants are more likely to have more frequent seizures. Some mothers carrying females have no seizures at all while pregnant.

○ Excessive vomiting of early pregnancy may be associated with increased seizure rates. This may be because anticonvulsant medicine can't be kept down.

○ For some reason, iron, vitamins D and K, and folic acid deficiency are more pronounced and severe in pregnant epileptics. The regular prenatal supplements of vitamins and minerals should manage all but the vitamin K needs. Authorities generally advise extra vitamin K administration, particularly toward the end of pregnancy. This supplemental K helps prevent internal hemorrhage in the newborn, a common cause of infant loss in epileptic mothers.

○ Unfortunately, the rate of congenital anomalies is greater when pregnancy is associated with epilepsy. Usually, such defects are the midline fusion type (harelip, cleft palate), but there are others. Whether this is a genetic factor or the result of anticonvulsant medications is not yet firmly established. Evidence linking some of the drugs used to control epilepsy with birth defects is becoming clearer. Your obstetrician will help you resolve your medication fears. One thing is clear: If convulsions persist or increase during pregnancy, your medications must be taken. Status epilepticus (constant uncontrolled seizures) must be avoided at all costs.

## THYROID DISORDERS

Everyone surely knows by now that the thyroid gland is the body thermostat. It controls the rate at which we burn fuel. *Hypo*thyroidism exists when we burn fuel too slowly, *hyper*thyroidism when we burn it too fast.

### Hypothyroidism

This condition may be caused by thyroid removal for cancer or for a number of other disorders. Hypothyroidism may also occur spontaneously in what was a previously healthy gland. Untreated, the condition shows itself by lassitude, tissue swelling, cold intolerance, weight gain, menstrual disturbances, and many other symptoms. If pregnancy takes place—and it is not easy—there is a much higher incidence of abortion, intrauterine fetal death, and congenital malformation. Fortunately, hypothyroidism is easy to detect and manage with modern laboratory procedures.

Hypothyroid patients should have their thyroid medication stabilized before trying to conceive. Close monitoring is necessary as pregnancy advances since at least one in four mothers require thyroid medication adjustment. With such care the fetal outcome is as good as any other primelife pregnancy and the infants are born with normal thyroid function.

## Hyperthyroidism

The motor is running too fast and the body becomes over-heated and overworked. For the 1 primelife mother in 2000 who has this disorder the common signs are sweating, nervousness, heat intolerance, heart palpitations, and increased appetite combined with weight loss. Unfortunately, some of these symptoms are also present in a normal early pregnancy and may cause some diagnostic confusion. Here is some more information:

○ There are many causes of hyperthyroidism. Even a certain abnormal placental disorder (hydatidiform mole; see Placenta, pages 113–14) can produce the disorder in early pregnancy.

○ Untreated, hyperthyroidism increases the risk of hypertension of pregnancy, increased perinatal mortality, and low birth weight infants.

○ The treatment during pregnancy may consist of partial thyroid removal or, difficult to explain, a combination of anti-thyroid and thyroid drugs.

○ Temporary thyroid disturbances may be found in the newborn children of hyperthyroid mothers, even those under treatment. Such disturbances are almost always short-lived. Very rarely, newborn thyrotoxicosis (toxic hyperthyroidism) may beset such an infant and with the potential for serious consequences. The child's symptoms may last as long as one year.

## AIDS

This disastrous import from abroad was first diagnosed in the United States in 1978. It first hit the medical press in 1981 and then the sensational press, where it has taken up permanent residence, a few hours later. And it's a sensational disorder with more medical and social implications than anything since we exported syphilis to Europe in the fourteenth century.

AIDS is caused by a retrovirus called HTLV III and is most commonly found in homosexual men (75 percent), intravenous drug abusers (20 percent), hemophiliacs (1 percent), recipients of blood transfusions containing the virus, and certain other uncommon sources.

Women may get the virus from men by anal (the most likely), vaginal, or oral sex. They may also get it from sharing needles with infected friends at drug parties. They may also become infected with the virus in certain occupations—a lab technician, for example, whose skin may be pierced by infected blood. Once the virus is living in their bodies they soon become sero-positive and thus react to the new blood test but they still may not get the full-blown clinically recognizable disease called AIDS. Even so, they can transmit the disease to others and to their intrauterine babes.

AIDS has thus become an obstetrical problem. Already, three maternal deaths from AIDS have been reported and many infants have been born with the disease, which can be transmitted to them in the uterus or at the time of birth or while breast feeding.

Here is a plan to follow:

○ While there are specific blood tests for AIDS, it is as yet not cost-effective to screen all pregnant women. Until it is, your obstetrician will test you only if you fit into the high-risk categories listed earlier or if you have specific symptoms of the disease or if you request a test.

○ Avoid occupations that might innocently expose you to the AIDS virus. This includes but is not limited to clinical laboratories, dental work, autopsy and mortician procedures, and work in certain custodial institutions.

○ Be continent in your sexual life. Avoid anal sex, which is not advisable during pregnancy anyway. Insist on condom protection if you are unsure about your mate.

○ Don't take drugs. Also, don't share razors, or even a toothbrush.

○ If you have a sero-positive blood test and are not pregnant, by all means avoid conceiving either until the test is proven wrong or until it becomes negative, which, thank God, can happen. Many women exposed to the disease and who become sero-positive can fight off the virus and become free of it and of the potential for getting the disease and passing it on.

# SURGICAL COMPLICATIONS OF PREGNANCY

Most surgery is tolerated very well by pregnant women, but unborn children often do not tolerate their mother's surgery very well. Even with the highest quality of care before, during, and after surgery, premature labor or intrauterine fetal loss are not uncommon companions of major surgical procedures during pregnancy.

Recognizing these facts, surgery in pregnancy is limited to two categories, traumatic and emergency. Elective surgical procedures are best avoided.

## Traumatic surgery

Almost 10 percent of all pregnant women sustain a traumatic injury of some sort. The majority of these injuries take place in an automobile or being propelled out of one. The rest happen around the house, usually in the bathroom or the kitchen. Physical abuse accounts for a few as do job-related accidents. Many traumatic injuries require surgical correction.

Pregnancy complicates traumatic surgical problems in that some of the common signs of internal injuries may be masked by pregnancy and may lead to diagnostic confusion. Any surgical procedures and any medications or anesthetics to be used must take the second life into account.

Generally, unless corrective surgical procedures involve opening the abdomen or the chest wall, and provided adequate oxygenation is supplied continuously, the infants fare well. In some instances, drugs to suppress uterine contractions may have to be used. Monitoring, where available, is continuous.

Other than trauma, the most likely acute surgical procedures are appendix, gallbladder, neoplastic surgery—the cervix, the ovaries, the breasts, and the skin (melanomas)—and heart surgery—coronary bypass, aneurysm repair, valve replacement or repair, and so forth.

Many other surgical procedures are less commonly performed during pregnancy. Even organ transplants can be managed (with great difficulty) when the mother's life is threatened. A *repeat* liver transplant during pregnancy has just been reported. In these situations the fetal risks are almost unsurmountable, yet the alternative is worse.

Primelife mothers are somewhat more likely to face some of the surgical complications listed above simply because they are at a time in life when precipitating factors are more likely to be present. Again, the maternal outcome is generally good, as good as anyone else's. The fetal outcome is improving.

## THE REGIONALIZATION OF MATERNAL CARE

The great advances in maternal care have been accompanied by the development of exotic and expensive equipment housed in an expensive environment and the creation of two medical subspecialties to manage mothers and infants brought to this environment for care. They are:

○ Neonatology. This specialty creates superpediatricians who live and work between the delivery room and their intensive-care nurseries. Called neonatologists, they are generally consulted about their anticipated high-risk infant charges, days, weeks, and even months before delivery is anticipated. Sometimes, however, they receive an unexpected one-pound infant with no prior warning at all! These specialists are consummately skilled in resuscitation of the newborn at delivery as well as the continuing care in their intensive-care nurseries. Further, they manage high-risk infants driven or flown in from satellite areas. (See below.)

○ Perinatology. This is the specialty for superobstetricians who devote their time to high-risk pregnancies. Perinatologists are also called maternal-fetal medicine specialists. They have the dubious honor of having to know all about obstetrics, general medicine, and fetal growth and development.

As these highly specialized maternity suites began to develop with their skilled subspecialists, it soon became clear that every hospital in the United States could not sustain the expense involved in supporting such exotic units, thus denying the best of care to high-risk mothers and infants in large areas of our country. Rather than allow this to happen, the obstetrical community, led by the American College of Obstetricians and Gynecologists, developed a national system of regionalized maternal and neonatal care. This system is in place and operating throughout virtually all of this country.

The whole country has been divided into geographically logical areas. Centrally located in each area, there lies a class III (or tertiary care) unit, usually, but not always, in a university medical center setting. A tertiary center contains all the equipment and support staff to manage the most critical high-risk maternal-fetal situation.

Surrounding the tertiary center are many hospitals with class II and I designations. Class II hospitals have maternity units that can manage normal deliveries and most cesarian sections. Maternity units in class I hospitals perform normal vaginal deliveries, but generally will not do cesarian sections unless a life-threatening situation exists that allows no time for patient transfer.

These designations are of course not hard and fast. Situations vary throughout our nation that require flexible applications of these guidelines. But they are the guidelines and we have established them to protect high-risk mothers and infants and to provide them with optimal care.

It is preferable for a primelife mother to avail herself of a tertiary center. Again, this is not always physically or geographically possible. However, each network has instant telecommunications among all units in the network for consultation and advice as well as to monitor interpretation and each has automobile or helicopter transport systems to bring mother and/or infant to the tertiary center.

In 1975, the Robert Wood Johnson Foundation provided $17.6 million to help establish and support for five years eight regionalization programs in diverse areas of the United States. Their goal was not only to help establish regionalization of maternal care, but further, to collect statistics that would reflect if such type of care actually promoted fetal and maternal well-being. The report of this experiment, published recently, indicated that the improved services for high-risk pregnancies resulted in significantly greater fetal salvage. Not only that:

    ° There was no increase in the pool of disabled children at one year of age. In other words, the level III units were not only saving little lives, they were saving healthy little lives.

○ There was an equally encouraging salvage at the other tertiary centers that were not in the program, but which were used as controls to establish validity to the studies. In other words, all others and self-sustaining tertiary centers were doing about as well.

○ Local and state governments in the eight test areas were equally impressed and continued to support the centers once the grant money was gone.

Thus, regionalization is a fact of American obstetrical life, and a blessing to many disadvantaged mothers and infants as well as to all mothers bearing children who, early or late in their pregnancy, must also bear an added risk for themselves or their beloved passenger.

○○○○○○○○○○○○ **THINGS TO THINK ABOUT** ○○○○○○○○○○○○

Sir Frederick Grant Best was born close to my birthplace in Ontario, Canada, but preceded me by many years. He became a physician and fought along with my father through all of World War I, returning afterward to Ontario to practice private medicine. His urge to do research interfered with his private career and so he moved to the University Medical School at Toronto where, during the year of my birth (1922) and about 150 miles away, he discovered insulin. His great contribution was instantly recognized, so that the very next year he was awarded the Nobel prize in medicine. Many other great awards, degrees, and honors were later bestowed upon him, including his knighthood. His findings, of course, revolutionized the treatment and survival of diabetics.

Sadly, he perished in the crash of a light aircraft in 1941, much younger than the new life expectancy that he had created for diabetics.

○○○○○○○

The total annual spending for all reproductive care, obstetrical care, and care of the newborn infant, including its first year of life, represents 5.5 percent of our total health care spending. By contrast 10 percent of all health care dollars were spent on persons in their last year of life and 33 percent went to those over sixty-five. Not to deny the senior citizen (of which I am one) or the moribund citizen (of which I am, thank God, not yet) any of their needs, but perhaps we have our medical priorities out of balance.

○ ○ ○ ○ ○ ○ ○

Heart transplant citizens can live relatively normal lives after their surgery. A forty-five-year-old Englishman named Brian Price recently completed the Boston marathon some fifteen months after his heart replacement surgery! No case is yet reported of a woman delivering a child after a heart transplant, but it is only a matter of time. As you know, many cases of successful pregnancy following kidney transplants are now recorded in the medical literature.

○ ○ ○ ○ ○ ○ ○

Exposure to viral infections while in the uterus may protect some infants against future disease, but increase the risk for others. Exposure to the herpes virus in utero, for example, increases a child's risk of future cancer, while exposure to mumps increases the risk of future diabetes. On the other hand, infants exposed to chicken pox while in utero have significantly less disorders of the skin and central nervous system. And everyone is or should be aware of the tragic effects of intrauterine exposure to rubella (German measles).

○ ○ ○ ○ ○ ○ ○

Macrosomia (birth weights in excess of 4500 grams—about ten pounds) is a complication of pregnancies that are associated with either maternal diabetes, obesity, or postmaturity. Such large infants are almost always male (over 70 percent), are delivered with much greater difficulty and with a greater incidence of birth injury, have lower Apgar scores, and greater fetal mortality. Bigger is not always better.

○ ○ ○ ○ ○ ○ ○

The common cold, which frequently attacks and tends to linger with pregnant women, is caused by at least six different kinds of rhinoviruses, and there may be others. The reservoir appears to be in children and when they return to school in the fall, they tend to accumulate different strains of the rhinovirus from old friends and then bring the new ones home to their own family. Thus, the cold season seems to start in the fall and is supposed to be related to chills and cold weather. This is not so. It starts with school. Another misconception is that a cold is spread by droplet infection carried in the air. Not so. The vast majority of colds are spread by hand contact either directly with an infected person or by touching something they have touched. So you know what to do.

There is no treatment on the horizon for colds. A tissue maker tried to market a disposable tissue impregnated with a chemical which absolutely reduced the spread of colds by a very significant amount. For some unknown reason the product didn't sell as well as expected and it is now being reevaluated. Sir William Osler, a famous physician of the past, probably had the best remedy of all: "Go to bed. Put a hat on the bedpost. Drink whiskey till you see two hats!"

Don't try it while you are pregnant.

○○○○○○○

Parenteral feeding in obstetrics. Intravenous feedings can sustain life for prolonged periods of time in a variety of medical conditions that prevent oral food intake. A recent study reports upon ten obstetrical patients who were fed and hydrated totally for as long as forty-seven days by the intravenous (parenteral) route. The individual needs for such therapy varied from severe vomiting to leukemia. All infants survived and were within normal birth weight ranges.

○○○○○○○○○○○○○○○○○○○○○○○○○○○○○○○○○○○○○○○○○○

○ 8 ○

# Assessment of Pregnancy Health in the Early Months

The recent advances in technological assessment of pregnancy and its well-being have taken place so rapidly and are advancing so quickly that it is almost impossible to establish a cutoff point in order to start describing and delineating all the available techniques and what they yield. The field of obstetrics, which has been until recently a specialty derived from observation and judgment, a stethescope, and a pair of forceps, has become an integrated circuit that cannot function without the backup support of a technical array. This is an exposition of the technical methods that are now, or soon will be, available to help us through the early months of a primelife pregnancy. None of these techniques are sunk in concrete, and indeed, they are constantly changing and being improved.

## BETA HCG

In the first chapter of this book, human chorionic gonadotropin (HCG) was identified as coming from the fetal placental tissue, specifically the chorion. This hormone appears almost immediately after fertilization and is detectable before the first missed period. The beta HCG fraction is a very reliable and specific component of the HCG complex. HCG, including beta, rises at a constant rate, doubling every other day in a normal pregnancy until

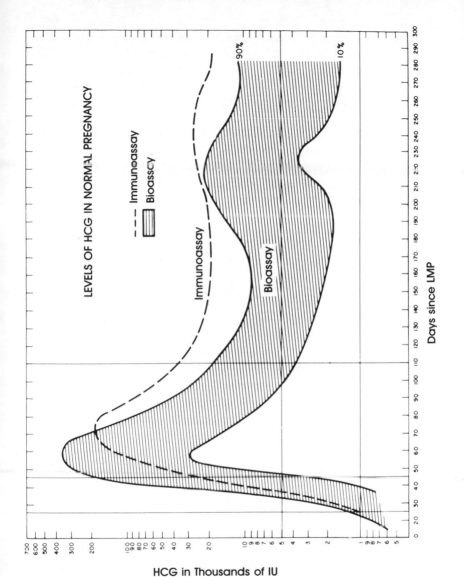

LEVELS OF HCG IN NORMAL PREGNANCY

- - - Immunoassay

||||| Bioassay

Immunoassay

Bioassay

90%

10%

HCG in Thousands of IU

Days since LMP

the seventieth day or thereabouts. Thereafter, the level falls gradually but will be present till term. See the graph on page 245.

Because these HCG levels are accurate and predictable, it has become possible not only to establish a pregnancy existence at a very early point but, further, to monitor the health of that pregnancy by plotting HCG levels. A decreasing value might very well signal a pregnancy in jeopardy and might further indicate the presence of an ectopic. Such test results, of course, must be interpreted in concert with other findings and by an expert.

Beta HCG testing is generally available everywhere in the United States. The cost is high but the eventual savings in time, pain, heartache, and other complications makes it very reasonable indeed.

## ULTRASOUND

Of all the technical procedures that have ever influenced obstetrics there is nothing that remotely compares to ultrasound. Now, I grant you, if you say that the introduction of sterile technique into the birth rooms during the germ theory revolution or the advent of blood transfusions are technological discoveries—and I suppose they are—then ultrasound may not be the greatest thing ever to come to the aid of pregnant women. After all, more women have died over the ages from puerperal sepsis (childbed fever) and from hemorrhage than have all the soldiers in all the wars from the beginning of time. Even so, little else in the field of technology can compare to ultrasound.

Fundamentally, medical ultrasound functions by means of echoes produced when a mechanical sound wave strikes internal tissues of different densities. To start it all off, a device in the ultrasound machine transforms electrical energy to sound energy (moving at 1540 meters per second), which penetrates tissues through a transducer device that is held against the skin. Different tissue densities return the echoes at different rates and in different amounts. The sound echoes thus generated return to the transducer and thence to the machine where they are converted back to electrical energy, which is itself converted to meaningful pictures on a screen.

From here on it gets very complicated. Some transducers send intermittent signals and wait for echo returns; some send constant signals from one area, receiving the echoes in another. Some are arranged to give better resolution of objects on different planes and others to display wider areas on the same plane. Thus, different modes of transmission supply different information about the tissues being examined. But the real breakthrough in sophisticated ultrasound has been the development of real-time imaging. Thus, we can see, live, dynamic displays of moving structures. We can see our unborn child moving, grimacing, clenching its fist, sucking its thumb, sticking out its tongue, swallowing amniotic fluid, and even emptying its bladder. We can see blood coursing through the placenta and umbilical vessels, see the heart beating as the various heart chambers contract and relax. And you can see it too. The ultrasonographers are happy to share the screen with you.

Most authorities in other countries recommend routine ultrasound scrutiny during pregnancy. In this country, routine screening has not been advised by national wisdom committees, which hold that the procedure is safe but not cost-effective. Probably that decision will soon be reversed. Some fifteen years of continuous and close scrutiny has failed to reveal the slightest evidence of fetal harm from single or repeated ultrasound exposures.

Standard and simple ultrasound procedures are often carried out in your obstetrician's office. More complicated examinations—the biophysical profile, for instance—requires a level II ultrasound setting (see pages 259–60). No matter, your involvement is the same. You are asked to drink water until you feel your back teeth are floating. Your bladder thus filled serves as a marker for the delineation of other organs. Your lower abdomen is coated with a cold clear cream, which serves to exclude air between you and the soon-to-be-applied transducer. This device looks like a long metal brush without any bristles. It sends the sound signals and receives the returning echoes and further reminds you of your full bladder. While the ultrasonographer scans your abdomen, you can join in the observation of incredible and fascinating fetal activity. Sadly, there are times when fetal problems are thus displayed, but most often, this is not the case and the pictures are very rewarding. Other than the full bladder, there are no discomforts associated with ultrasound procedures and, again, they are safe.

In early pregnancy monitoring ultrasound can determine:

○ That pregnancy exists. About the fifth or sixth week, the fetal sac appears as a little bubble in the uterine cavity and shortly thereafter a tiny nub can be seen somewhere on the rim of that bubble. That is the fetal pole. Somewhere around the seventh week the fetal heart can actually be seen to be beating in that fetal pole, an amazing sight indeed. These are all *proof positive* that a living pregnancy exists in the uterus.

○ The duration of pregnancy. Many times the actual duration of pregnancy is an important piece of information. Using the above guidelines and some other ultrasound refinements, accurate dating is possible. So if the last menstrual period is unknown or the pregnancy does not conform to the last menstrual period, ultrasound will supply the answer. In primelife pregnancies the exact duration of pregnancy may be of great importance. Growth retardation in late pregnancy is more common here for a number of reasons (see pages 133–34). If the exact dating of the pregnancy has been available all along then there is less chance for error in establishing the diagnosis of IUGR.

○ The exact location of pregnancy. It is clear that when the pregnancy is seen in the uterine cavity it is where it belongs. If, on the other hand, pregnancy is known to exist but the uterus is empty by ultrasound, things are not well. The fetal sac should then appear on the screen in one tube or another and diagnosis of an ectopic has been confirmed. It is not as simple as it sounds, but ultrasound is of great help in locating pregnancies exactly.

○ The health of an early pregnancy. If there is any reason to suspect the health and continued growth of a pregnancy it can be clearly demonstrated by an ultrasound study. An empty fetal sac or one containing a disintegrated embryo with no heartbeat are clear signs of disaster and prevents days, even weeks, of agonizing. On the other hand, increasing fetal development with an active heartbeat all augur well for the pregnancy.

○ The number of pregnancies present. The diagnosis of twins and more by this type of study must be handled with great care in early pregnancy. Sacs can be missed and false sacs can be counted so in the event that there is any doubt, a repeat study should be made later on.

Ultrasound can also be used:

○ To follow up AFP studies (see page 253). If a maternal AFP study is abnormal, then an ultrasound is indicated to display fetal spinal integrity or lack of it.

○ To identify the amniotic sac location (see page 251).

Mind you, these are nowhere near all the uses for ultrasound in the study of early pregnancy health—or illness.

## GENETICS

Most everyone over thirty-five already knows that each cell in the human body contains within its nucleus twenty-three paired chromosomes, twenty-two matching autosomes and a pair of sex chromosomes. Each chromosome, which is itself a long strand of protein, carries a great number of little dots matching a somewhat similar dot on its paired mate. These dots are genes and are responsible for our inherited characteristics. Most of them have been mapped like the stars, and their precise location and responsibilities are known. Sex chromosomes are known as X and Y, a male being XY and a female XX. At maturation of spermatozoa, the chromosome pairs separate and each goes their own way into a sperm head. Thus there are in each mature sperm head twenty-two unpaired autosomes and either an X or a Y sex chromosome. Got it? Now a mature unfertilized egg when it leaves the ovary also has twenty-two unpaired autosomes plus one sex chromosome, always an X. At the act of fertilization, the chromosomes pair up. If the sperm head contains a Y, then it's another damned boy, and if it contains an X, well, then, it is a little girl.

Chromosomes can be damaged by radiation and some chemicals. Freezing will not damage them and frozen embryos can be restored. As we get older, chromosomes tend to get sticky, particularly in some locations along their strands. Thus incomplete and abnormal separations may take place in the maturing egg or sperm and the resultant union at fertilization can give us real problems. One of these is Down's syndrome, once called mongolism. Down's syndrome occurs with increasing frequency after thirty-five. Thus, the rate between thirty-five and forty is 1 in 250 births, forty to forty-five, 1 in 100, forty-five and up, 1 in 40.

Finally, there are a number of inherited disorders that will pass from generation to generation. Some of them are on autosomes (Tay-Sachs disease, for instance) and some are sex chromosome–linked (hemophilia). Some eighty disorders of such a nature can be identified by amniocentesis and genetic analysis.

## GENETIC COUNSELING

When one suspects that the likelihood of a genetic disorder is increased in a particular pregnancy because of age, familial history, or radiation or toxic exposure, then genetic counseling and amniocentesis is recommended.

Here is how it works. A geneticist or the equivalent in training will counsel on the yield from amniocentesis and tissue culture and will predict the chances of occurrence of the defect for which the study is being contemplated. Moreover, during the counseling at some point the risks of the proposed procedure to both mother and fetus will be clearly delineated. Thus at the end of the conference the yield and the risks have been clearly defined. If at this point the mother cannot accept the possibility of a therapeutic abortion should the cultures reveal a defect, the study is discontinued and everybody signs documents. If, on the other hand, abortion is acceptable, then amniocentesis is arranged.

Prior to the actual amniocentesis an ultrasound examination is begun. Most often this is in or around the fifteenth week of pregnancy. Before that time there is too little amniotic fluid and after the fifteenth week the results may come in too late for therapeutic pregnancy termination.

## AMNIOCENTESIS

Two sacs surround the fetus, an outer chorion (remember?) and an inner amnion. Both layers are closely approximated. Inside the amnion is fluid, amniotic fluid, a liquid in constant and complex circulation. It increases from a few drops at the beginning to over a quart at full term but is always changing and circulating. Removal of samples of this fluid offers a startling array of information throughout pregnancy, but at this time we want it for biochemical analysis and for the culture of fetal cells that have slipped away from the fetus and circulate in it.

The operator now looks at the ultrasound display and sees where the amniotic sac is located. Under local anesthesia, a needle is inserted through the maternal abdomen into the uterus and into the amniotic sac, and a measured amount of fluid is withdrawn. Some of the yield is used for a variety of biochemical tests (see AFP, page 253, for instance) and the rest is sent for tissue culture which may take several weeks. This may fail and require, God forbid, a repeat amniocentesis.

Should the amniocentesis demonstrate that the unwanted defect is indeed present, then arrangements must be made to carry out the therapeutic termination of that pregnancy. Usually the cultures take two to three weeks to harvest and are virtually 100 percent correct in the information that they yield, which incidentally includes the sex.

Although the procedure is relatively painless (according to those submitting to it), there are some hazards that accompany it which need to be defined.

○ Failure. As noted above, the culture may not grow and may have to be repeated.

There may even be insufficient fluid present to supply an adequate sample and the distance from the skin to the sac may be too great to allow penetration (obesity).

The placenta may be in such a location as to prevent safe penetration. Newer techniques may have partially resolved that problem.

○ Rh reactions may occur. Minute amounts of fetal blood may get into the maternal circulation. If the mother is Rh negative and the fetus is Rh positive, sensitization might take place (see pages 120–23). Thus all Rh negative mothers receive Rh vaccine after an amniocentesis. This is quite safe.

Although amniocentesis is a very commonly performed procedure, it is generally performed only at tertiary care obstetricial centers (see pages 240–41). Their locations are well known to all practicing obstetricians.

The cost of amniocentesis and genetic counseling varies from one part of our country to another but is usually in the $800 to $1000 range. Some insurance policies cover the procedure and some countries with national health plans pay for the whole thing. However, they are not always obtainable at any price in those countries. Finally, there are other uses for amniocentesis in later pregnancy and they will be described in the next chapter.

## CHORIONIC VILLI SAMPLING

Recently the obstetrical literature from other countries— China, Great Britain, and Italy, in particular—has been flooded with information on a bold new technique that will perhaps replace early amniocentesis for our genetic testing. Called chorionic villi sampling (CVS), the procedure is based upon the fact that the chorionic membrane is covered in early pregnancy with the chorionic villi (remember early pregnancy testing and HCG). These spongelike villi gradually recede from the membrane except in the one area where they form the embedding placenta. But until they do, they are available for biopsy in the uterine cavity. Ultrasound is used to direct a probe through the cervix into the uterus and the biopsy is taken. The chorionic villi are, of course, fetal cells, and as such, carry all the information needed for genetic and biochemical studies. The procedure has several real advantages:

   ° It can be done early—from six to twelve weeks but usually the ninth week.

   ° The tests are completed within a day or so after the procedure, allowing very early termination if indicated.

   ° The procedure is less hazardous to the mother and, if uncomplicated, the amniotic sac is not invaded.

   ° It will be less expensive.

There are, however, some real disadvantages:

   ° It is still experimental and approved in this country at only a few institutions as an experimental procedure.

- There is more fetal loss at this point, perhaps two times greater than with amniocentesis. This will continue to decrease as techniques and skills improve.

- There is more danger of contamination with maternal cells so that the results might not be accurate.

- As with all complicated procedures, there is the ever-present risk of failure.

- It will not detect neural tube defects, thus an AFP (see below) is necessary.

- An Rh vaccine must be given to Rh negative women following this procedure.

As time goes on you will read more and more about CVS, and it is very likely that it, or something close to it, will eventually replace amniocentesis.

## ALPHA FETOPROTEIN (AFP)

Early in pregnancy, the fetus secretes this protein in the area of the spinal canal as the canal, cord, and brain are developed. When the spinal canal and brain are completely enclosed, as they should be by the end of the first trimester, AFP should no longer be spilled out in any significant amount and therefore none of it escapes into the maternal circulation. If it does, then there may be a defect in the spinal closure, or worse. Disorders such as spina bifida at one end to a monstrous deformity of the head at the other may be present.

So it is that testing the maternal serum for AFP at about the fifteenth week is gradually becoming a routine test procedure. The testing material is available everywhere in this country. If an abnormally high test result is obtained, then an ultrasound examination is indicated. The test may be elevated even though everything appears normal. In that case, it will be repeated and the pregnancy watched very closely. Incidentally, an AFP determination is always, or almost always, done at amniocentesis.

## MANAGING THE TORCH COMPLEX

Chapter Four describes the TORCH complex. You may recall that the word *TORCH* is a symbol for a number of unrelated infectious disorders that can have profound effects on pregnancy. Many times these diverse infections will follow common pathways in their destructive attacks on pregnancy. Thus the actual culprit may not be identified or identifiable.

Remember, then, that TORCH stands for:

**T** — Toxoplasmosis

**O** — Others: hepatitis B, Beta streptoccocus, influenza, mumps, varicella (chicken pox), and others

**R** — Rubella (German measles)

**C** — Cytomegalovirus (CMV)

**H** — Herpes virus II

Unfortunately, there are constant additions to this complex of viral and bacterial disorders that can seriously hamper pregnancy, but the main offenders are listed above.

What can be done?

In early pregnancy, obstetricians usually test for the presence of toxoplasmosis and rubella titers as part of routine blood work. Soon, CMV will also have an available blood test in the prenatal profile. In the event of an unexplained febrile illness during pregnancy, changes in these titers yield important information and give us an opportunity to determine if one of these viruses has indeed attacked the maternal host and perhaps the child. Thus, an alert is issued to watch for potential fetal complications during pregnancy and after birth. We can now culture throughout early (and late) pregnancy for herpes II and for Beta streptoccocus. A vaccine is now available to protect mothers from hepatitis B.

○○○○○○○○○○○○○ **THINGS TO THINK ABOUT** ○○○○○○○○○○○○○○

In a recent study of seventy-five high-risk pregnancies conducted by D. M. Wass, et al., in the *Australian and New Zealand Journal of Obstetrics and Gynecology,* all mothers were offered prenatal genetic diagnosis—either amniocentesis, which yields findings at nineteen to twenty weeks, or chorionic villi sampling, which yields findings at six to eleven weeks of pregnancy. Although each patient was advised that the risk of abortion was about five times greater with CVS, fifty of them accepted that procedure as the one of choice. The wait time made the difference.

○ ○ ○ ○ ○ ○ ○

In regards to the above findings, many of us in the profession fail to realize the anxiety that accompanies the twenty days or so between amniocentesis and the results. All of these pregnancies are, after all, dearly wanted, else the testing would not be submitted to. Although the quality and strength of attachment grows more strongly in the later trimesters, a great deal of fantasizing and even bonding develops from the moment of conceptual knowledge. The waiting period, then, is an important psychological time that needs to be dealt with. It may be compressed into a few hours by the newer techniques, but it still must be dealt with.

○ ○ ○ ○ ○ ○ ○

Circadian cycles in the fetal urinary bladder during pregnancy have been observed by ultrasound. It has been demonstrated that the fetal bladder fills very slowly from midnight to 6:00 A.M. No changes occur because of daylight saving time, *but* time zone changes are observed.

○ ○ ○ ○ ○ ○ ○

In regards to Baby Doe regulations, the federal government has maintained that it has the right to interfere in the management of grossly deformed, disadvantaged, or barely viable infants if in its infinite wisdom it feels that the specialists who have devoted their lives to such infants are giving less than maximum effort to sustain them. They even installed hot lines in hospital intensive-care nurseries so that anyone could call Washington direct and blow the whistle on backsliders.

Devoted neonatologists, pediatricians, perinatologists, obstetricians, medical societies, and many caring people were furious, not only at the unwarranted intrusion, but at what the intrusion implied.

On June 9, 1986, the Supreme Court forbade the federal government to interfere further in the management of these infants.

○ ○ ○ ○ ○ ○ ○

Some facts about birth defects:

- As mentioned earlier, birth defects are gradually increasing worldwide. No one knows why.

- Heart defects are increasing most rapidly, spinal defects are decreasing, and cleft palate, cystic kidneys, clubfoot, and Down's syndrome remain about the same.

- Exposure to a teratogen of any sort in the first two weeks of pregnancy generally results in a spontaneous abortion rather than a defective infant.

- The most critical time for defect formation is after the second week of actual pregnancy and before the tenth. That would be from the fourth to the twelfth week, counting from the last menstrual period.

- Again, counting from the actual day of conception, the most critical period of central nervous system development is the third to sixth week; of the heart, from 3.5 to 6.5 weeks; the eyes, 3.5 to 8.5 weeks.

- Abortion is usually recommended for women exposed to over ten rads of radiation in early pregnancy. Rads are a unit of x-ray activity.

- In 1984, congential anomalies were the fifth leading cause of years of potential life lost before age sixty-five. They accounted for 684,000 years of potential life lost.

○ ○ ○ ○ ○ ○ ○ ○ ○ ○ ○ ○ ○ ○ ○ ○ ○ ○ ○ ○ ○ ○ ○ ○ ○ ○ ○ ○ ○ ○ ○ ○ ○ ○ ○ ○ ○ ○ ○ ○ ○ ○ ○ ○ ○

o ⑨ o

# Assessment of Pregnancy Health in the Later Months

This chapter concerns itself with methods of monitoring fetal state as pregnancy advances upon term and maturity. True fetal state is dependent upon the levels and distribution of central nervous system energy. When all is going well for the fetus, the distribution of energy and stimuli to the rest of its developing body is quite adequate and all systems perform much like a marvelous intercompany computer system with a great mainframe that is never down. There is, however, a great deal of rhythmic control built into the fetal system. These are called biorhythms, and the longest such rhythm lasts twenty-five hours and exists from conception till death, which is one reason why we adults have difficulty adjusting to a twenty-four-hour day!

But to go on. There are many minor rhythms going on inside the major fetal biorhythm, one of which is the twenty- to forty-minute rest/sleep cycle observed in all human fetuses. At least 80 percent of fetal time is spent in sleep, and most of that is in REM (rapid eye movement) sleep. This has been documented very clearly by ultrasound. It is during REM sleep that a great deal of fetal brain organization is believed to be accomplished, and during this sleep, the brain shuts itself off *completely* from the external environment.

What does it all mean? To you and to me? Let's go back to the big analogy of the company computer. The fetal mainframe is constantly on—there is an eternal hum. At times, it is working furiously and at times resting but never, *ever* off. It sends signals to the body terminals and they send signals back. If the mainframe electricity is cut off, good-bye. If the electrical flow is uneven, bad data, bad instructions, bad results. The fetal brain, then, given adequate oxygen and glucose, supplies the energy in a rhythmic flow that makes the total system go and grow. Our monitoring efforts must tell us that the fetal brain is being supplied adequately and constantly with oxygen and glucose.

Further, our attempts to monitor fetal state must take into account the rhythmic nature of state. Thus, a healthy fetus may respond to external sound or abdominal palpation at one time, but during a period of REM sleep, may be totally unmoved and unmovable but still healthy. Our attempts to monitor fetal state in advancing pregnancy must take these variables of fetal rhythm and activity into account, as well as displaying the basic brain activity and responses.

Some interesting sidelights:

○ During fetal REM sleep (which is when adults dream; no one has any idea what fetuses do), the infant can be seen clenching its jaw, opening and closing its mouth, sticking out its tongue, and generally making faces.

○ Fetal activity and movements increase as the day progresses and, as any weary mother already knows, tends to peak about midnight.

○ Infants breathe most rapidly during the night and fill their bladders most rapidly in late afternoon.

## MORE ULTRASOUND

Much has been said of the application of ultrasound in all sections of this book. Too much cannot be said. It is difficult to imagine the proper management of pregnancy without this magnificent tool.

Ultrasound's role in early pregnancy management has already been explored. Now, in the third trimester, ultrasound can be used:

○ To determine placental location. An abnormal placental implant low in the uterus and lying over the cervix (placenta previa) can be readily detected.

° To determine abruptio placenta. Premature separation of a normally implanted placenta can be disastrous for both mother and child. Usually it is seen clearly on ultrasound.

° To estimate pregnancy duration when the menstrual dates and other dating information is inadequate.

° To follow up observation of previously detected congenital malformations.

° As an adjunct to intrauterine manipulations such as fetoscopy (see page 273), intrauterine transfusion (see page 122), and late amniocentesis.

° To detect and follow intrauterine growth retardation (IUGR, see pages 133–34).

° As the biophysical profile (BPP). This important ultrasound procedure needs to be dealt with at length.

Clearly, we are concerned with fetal health and growth and development (state) throughout all of pregnancy. Further, we are infinitely concerned about fetal state in primelife pregnancies, pregnancies complicated by serious maternal illness, and pregnancies complicated by serious obstetrical disorders.

Since the fetus becomes more accessible and more nearly viable while the third trimester unfolds, our concern for fetal state reveals itself in the numerous tests, which we have brought on line during these critical weeks to tell us what we so dearly want to know: Fetus, how are you doing?

## Biophysical profile (BPP)

Of all the tests now available to us, the biophysical profile is probably the most important and the most revealing. This particular ultrasound determination requires a level II ultrasound clinic (see pages 240–41) and a skilled ultrasonographer. It is generally first obtained around the twenty-eighth week of pregnancy. Here is the data which is recorded:

° Fetal size is determined by measurements of critical diameters and bone lengths. From this data, an estimate of fetal age is made.

° The amount of amniotic fluid present. Too much or too little may signal problems.

° Placental age. Placentas get old and get arteriosclerosis; sometimes, with certain maternal disorders, they get too old too soon.

° Fetal breathing.

° Fetal heart rate and reactivity.

° Fetal body movements and tone (grasping, grimacing, etc.).

° Very recently and with state-of-the-art equipment, blood flow rates through the umbilical vessels. This is rapidly becoming a most important measurement.

All this accumulated data is assembled and a score is assigned, ten being perfect. A fetus entering the twenty-eighth week of pregnancy with a perfect ten or even close to it is in excellent state and the coming twelve weeks look good for it. This is not to suggest that no further BPPs or other tests of state will be in order as time goes on. Far from it. But a good BPP is a great way for a primelife fetus to enter the third trimester. The other side of the coin, a low BPP score, needs to be dealt with.

An unsatisfactory BPP indicates serious problems and dictates that very close observation accompanied by repeat BPPs and other tests of fetal health must be made. It also means a thorough review of maternal well-being and compliance. Moreover, an early delivery may be in the offing.

## Some more about ultrasound

° Soon, we will be able to detect over two thirds of all congenital anomalies by ultrasound. Almost that percentage is being detected now, and in many cases, intervention by means of medication or surgery can salvage some of these potentially healthy members of society before they are born.

° Sophisticated ultrasound measurement of umbilical blood flow rates may turn out to be the earliest method of detecting inadequate placental transfer, and thus the very onset of declining state.

° Fetal sex determination is virtually 90 percent possible now. If you can't see it, it's a girl!

° Magnetic resonance imaging is a new, fantastic, and apparently safe technique, which allows us to look at the inside of a body almost as clearly as the outside. MRI involves no ionizing radiation (like x-rays) and no known adverse maternal or fetal effects. Its only present drawbacks are its availability and its expense. Here are some of its advantages:

° The whole uterus, placenta, and fetus can be seen at one time.

° No shadows are cast as occurs with ultrasound.

° Physiological events can be witnessed in the placenta, allowing better determination of placental health.

° Possible disproportion between the fetal head and the maternal pelvis can be better visualized.

° Oligohydramnios (scant amniotic fluid) is more readily determined.

° As it becomes less expensive and more widely available, MRI will very clearly play a large role in obstetrical affairs.

° At this time the BPP accompanied by maternal self-assessment (see pages 269–70) represents the best way of monitoring fetal state.

## MONITORING FOR FETAL STRESS AND DISTRESS

When it became possible for doctors to manage pregnancy, methods for assessing fetal health soon emerged—nothing too sophisticated, mind you, but a step forward.

The most obvious, available, and measurable item was the fetal heart. And it is still, with some modern refinements. In the beginning, though, brave physicians would listen to the fetal heart by placing one ear or the other (depending, I guess, on which way they wanted to face!) on the maternal abdomen. After the twentieth week, the fetal heart could then—and can still—be heard very clearly. You obviously can't try this technique on yourself, but your unimpregnated coconspirator can—or anyone else you may relinquish your tummy to.

As time went on, physicians became more withdrawn from their patients and so they invented little hollow ear horns about eight inches long, which transmitted the fetal heart sounds reasonably well, and apparently, at a reasonable distance. Eventually, even this was too close and the stethoscope became the accepted way to listen to the heartbeat. Incidentally, very little was then noted about the fetal heart except whether it was beating or whether it wasn't. Not so today.

The fetal heart still remains the most accessible, easily monitored prognostic fetal organ. Because it reflects very quickly the fetal central nervous system state, it has become the marker for modern nonstress and stress testing.

In order to carry out such testing, a typical fetal-maternal monitor such as those used to follow labor is employed. These devices can monitor and record simultaneously both fetal heart rates and uterine contractions. Here are the physiological principles involved in heart rate testing:

○ Inadequate levels of oxygen and glucose to the fetal brain affect the central mainframe. And one of the first organs to reflect decreased central well-being is the fetal heart.

○ A healthy uterine-placental environment offers no stress to a fetus. It has regular sleep/wake episodes and reacts to external stimuli, such as noise or movement. Such reactions normally increase its heart rate.

○ An unfavorable uterine-placental environment will alter state adversely, and the fetal heart will now respond to activity in a sluggish way or not at all.

○ If the unfavorable environment escalates, the fetal heart rate will decline when stress is introduced, stress being introduced by the external production of uterine contractions using mechanisms to be described shortly.

○ In time, fetal stress will lead to fetal distress, just as continued adult stress will lead to adult distress. Both states should be avoided.

Basically, there are two types of monitoring, external and internal. Internal monitoring is used only during labor, while external monitoring is used both to follow labor and to perform fetal stress studies.

## External monitoring

External monitoring during labor requires fetal and uterine observations. These procedures carry no risks whatsoever.

○ Fetal heart rate. To obtain fetal heart rates through the abdominal and uterine walls, an ultrasound principle is employed. Pulsed high-frequency sound waves are transmitted from a small transducer applied to the abdominal wall over the area of clearest fetal heartbeat activity. The resultant echoes return to the abdominal transducer and are converted to electrical energy, which can be heard and also recorded on a continuous paper strip. (See the sample on page 264.) Each dot on the paper strip usually represents the average of three beats.

○ Uterine contractions. A famous physiologist, Dr. Sam Reynolds, was the first person to discover a reliable method of measuring uterine contractions through an intact abdominal wall. I had the honor of being his assistant in many of his early experiments. He developed a strain-gauge ring which, when fastened to the abdominal skin, recorded elliptical curve changes that accompanied uterine contractions. The same curvature changes occur along a length of thin wood when it is bent. These curvature changes, converted to electrical energy, could be recorded on continuous flow paper strips and indicated the duration and amplitude of uterine contractions as well as the interval between contractions. Modern methods of recording uterine contractions are still based upon the principles that Dr. Reynolds discovered. Thus, today we attach a sophisticated type of strain gauge to the abdominal wall when we want to measure and record uterine contractile activity in a noninvasive way. Placement of both fetal and uterine recording devices upon the abdomen are painless and harmless.

## Internal monitoring

Restricted to the laboring mother, internal observations of fetal health and uterine activity are certainly more accurate but not without some risk. Such risks must be weighed against the accurate information that internal monitoring displays.

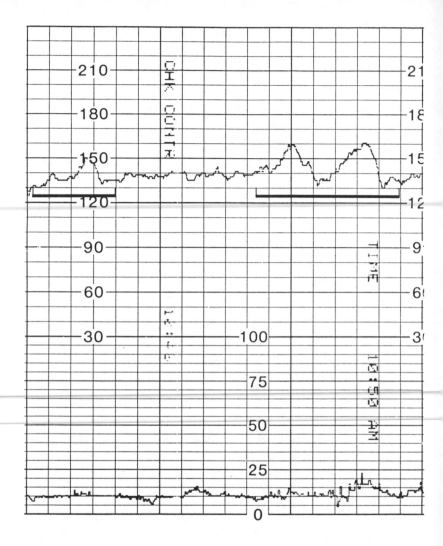

A monitor strip taken during a nonstress test. It is a reactive (normal) test, indicated by the rhythmic increases in fetal heart rate (marked with brackets) in the upper tracing. The lower tracing is of maternal uterine contractions, of which there is none.

○ Internal fetal monitoring. In order to get a direct, continuous, and accurate fetal electrocardiogram, an electrode is attached to the infant's scalp once it can be clearly felt during labor. Usually, the cervix has dilated several centimeters before such an attachment is possible. If the membranes have not previously ruptured, the attachment of a fetal electrode will surely accomplish it. Once attached and connected to our recording devices, we have a beat-by-beat display of the actual fetal cardiac activity and well-being as labor progresses. Scalp electrodes are used only during labor or after the membranes are ruptured spontaneously or artificially for whatever reason. Some risks are involved in the attachment of a fetal scalp electrode. The benefits most always outweigh the risks.

Scalp electrodes may soon transmit more information than just the fetal heart activity. Modern technology may soon be able to display the Ph of fetal blood on a continuing basis through the same single scalp application. The Ph of fetal blood is the single most valuable evidence of fetal health that we know of and such information, reliably presented, will mark a significant step forward in fetal protection during labor.

○ Internal uterine monitoring. Abdominal strain-gauge evaluation of uterine contractions, although very reliable, cannot assess the strength and tone of uterine contractions as accurately as a well-placed internal monitor. Again, such monitoring activity is restricted to active labor, and, usually, special circumstances.

Once the cervix is sufficiently dilated, a plastic catheter is guided into the uterine cavity to lie in its middle to upper areas. Such a catheter, connected to a closed fluid column, measures not only uterine contractions and their frequency but also the force and strength of such contractions with accuracy not achieved externally. But note that the placental location must be clearly out of the way of the catheter and that internal uterine monitoring is restricted to active labor. Certain risks are involved with this procedure and they must be outweighed by the sensitivity of the information obtained.

## New types of fetal monitoring

Here are two new types of fetal monitoring that are now under study and should be considered investigational:

    ° A lightweight portable monitor has been developed for home use. Attached to the maternal abdomen, it records uterine contractions which are telecommunicated to hospital interpretation centers. It is hoped that such devices can alert mothers at high risk for premature labor to the earliest indications of abnormal uterine activity.

    ° A startle test for the evaluation of fetal central nervous system state is also under investigation. During ultrasound surveillance, a hand held buzzer is placed against the maternal abdomen. The noise so produced can be heard by the fetus and its startle response observed. The response consists of head aversion, eye blinking, mouth opening, and other reactions. It has also been noted that a healthy fetus will react less vigorously to repeated sound stimulation—like an adult to a snooze alarm. Again, this test is still investigational in nature, but may join our armamentarium for intrauterine fetal monitoring.

## THE FETAL NONSTRESS TEST

Armed with information about fetal physiology and about the mechanisms of monitoring, a nonstress test should now have some meaning for you. Here basically is the rest:

    ° Using a stethoscope or some other transmitting device, the fetal heart is located at its maximal transmitting area on the maternal abdominal wall and an ultrasound transmitter is applied to that spot. The fetal heart can now be heard and recorded on a continuous paper strip.

    ° Typical nonstress recording can be obtained either in a labor suite or in your obstetrician's office. Usually, you will be lying flat and on your left side or lying back somewhat in a recliner.

    ° Observations and tracings of the fetal heart rate are observed for some minutes to develop a baseline pattern.

- Fetal heart rate patterns are now observed during wake periods and during external stimulation, if necessary. Normally, the heart accelerates during these episodes for a predictable period of time.

- Normal acceleration indicates a reactive nonstress test, a reassuring event. If acceleration does not take place, we have a nonreactive nonstress test, and further studies are in order.

## FETAL STRESS TESTING

These procedures are usually reserved to follow nonreactive nonstress testing but this is not always so. Stress testing involves efforts to put the fetus into a stressful environment. This is most usually accomplished by producing uterine contractions one way or another. During an active, intense uterine contraction, uterine and therefore placental circulation stops. In health, the placenta has an adequate reserve of oxygen and glucose to protect the fetus during this circulation shutdown. An aged or diseased placenta cannot always do so and thus some asphyxia occurs, state is disrupted, and distress signals go out from the mainframe to the terminals. Among other terminals, the heart is notified and it reacts.

### The oxytocin stress test

Known by other names (contraction stress test, oxytocin contraction test, etc.), this procedure is an extension of the nonstress test. Using the same monitor, a gauge is now placed on the abdomen which can record uterine contractions. Through an intravenous infusion, oxytocin (the pituitary substance, which can produce uterine contractions) is administered. Soon measurable uterine contractions occur. If the uterine-placental environment is healthy, there will be little or no change in the recorded fetal heart rate. If, on the other hand, placental reserves are inadequate, the FHR begins to decline toward the end of each contraction as oxygen runs out. This is called a positive stress test, and it indicates present or impending fetal distress. It also indicates some definitive treatment. See the sample on page 268.

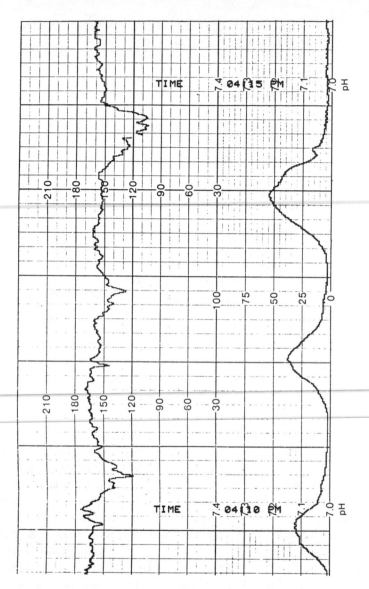

A monitor strip showing a reactive stress test. After each uterine contraction, produced either by oxytocin or by breast stimulation (see pages 267 and 269), there is a significant drop in the fetal heart rate. This indicates placental insufficiency and fetal stress.

## The breast stimulation test

Breast stimulation has long been known to induce uterine contractions. That is why, for instance, nursing will increase afterpains. Using this reflex principle, many investigators are now substituting breast stimulation for oxytocin to evoke uterine contractions. Let me anticipate morbid enquiry here by saying that the mother stimulates her own breasts to initiate the contractions. Once a contraction pattern is initiated, the test proceeds exactly as does the OCT above, and the interpretation is the same.

Some points about OCT and BST stress testing:

    ° These procedures are often best avoided when there has been a previous cesarian section or a history of premature labor. A BPP is perhaps a better alternative.

    ° Stress testing is probably a more reliable indicator of fetal distress than the nonstress test.

    ° The BST is simpler to perform and can be accomplished in an office setting.

    ° Mothers who react strongly to breast stimulation should avoid nipple preparation for nursing and should also avoid breast stimulation during foreplay.

## MATERNAL SELF-MONITORING

As an important adjunct to electronic monitoring, mothers are now regularly enlisted to observe and record fetal movements on a daily basis. Such recordings are usually initiated at the beginning of the third trimester. Primelife mothers are asked to record fetal movements during three preselected times daily. Those times vary, but usually include an early morning and late evening segment. Normally, at least three movement episodes are expected within a half hour's time. If not, the observation time may be extended. Fetal activity thus observed is recorded and reported at regular obstetrical visits. Your own obstetrician should be consulted at once should there be less than ten movements over a twelve-hour period of observation, no movements are encountered in the mornings, or your recordings reveal a pattern of declining fetal activity.

As I stated earlier, I believe that the combination of maternal self-monitoring and the biophysical profile offers us the best method of evaluating and following fetal health at this time, but times are changing rapidly.

## The frequency of monitoring

o Maternal self-monitoring is a daily event and this is one major reason why it is such a valuable test.

o Nonstress testing commonly takes place each week once it is begun. In certain situations involving serious obstetrical complications (a severe diabetic with a bad pregnancy history, for example), NST may be obtained every few days. They are perfectly safe, and since they are usually an office procedure, the cost is not great.

o The OCT and BST are likely to have been preceded by an NST which did not react properly. Sometimes, though, these challenge tests are used by themselves and without previous nonstress testing. Some observers feel they are much more sensitive, and so they bypass the NST. No matter what, once a stress test reveals evidence of fetal distress, it is time to intervene and to stop testing.

## MATERNAL BLOOD TESTS FOR FETAL STATE

In certain reproductive disorders, some evidence of fetal health can be obtained from maternal blood serum. For instance:

o Alpha fetoprotein (AFP) is becoming increasingly valuable as a screening test for fetal neural tube defects. (See page 253.)

o Estriol is an estrogen substance that is secreted by the placenta throughout pregnancy. The amounts produced are measurable and predictable, increasing regularly till near the end of pregnancy. As placental senescence approaches, estriol secretion decreases. Should early placental senescence take place (as in diabetes, malnutrition, or hypertensive cardiovascular disease), then maternal estriol levels will drop. Widely used in the past, estriol testing has been largely replaced by more available ultrasound and monitoring procedures.

○ Rh blood testing. When Rh incompatibility is a potential complicating factor, regular Coombs' tests are in order. This test measures the levels of circulating maternal Rh antibodies. Rising titers may indicate the need for early intervention in the pregnancy management.

○ Regular blood sugar levels are important in managing diabetic and gestational diabetic pregnancies. Moreover, a maternal blood test to demonstrate the presence of an unusual hemoglobin (hemoglobin C) is of great value in assessing any degree of prolonged and excessive blood sugar levels (hyperglycemia). HGB C determinations therefore represent an excellent way of monitoring insulin and dietary adequacy as well as maternal compliance. Most maternal diabetics are very disciplined in their personal medical control.

## AMNIOCENTESIS

The transabdominal withdrawal of amniotic fluid in late pregnancy is very safe and yields a variety of information about state. Under local anesthesia and with ultrasound guidance, amniocentesis is usually safe and relatively free of discomfort. Here are some things that amniocentesis reveals:

○ Fetal lung maturity. A variety of procedures are available that, by measuring certain components of amniotic fluid, can predict the degree of fetal lung maturity. Such information is of great value when early delivery is indicated for any reason. For instance, in managing severe hypertension of pregnancy that is not responsive to conservative therapy, emptying the uterus before full term may be necessary. The degree of fetal lung maturity is an important consideration in the timing of such a delivery. Medications are available to help speed up fetal lung maturation under such circumstances, but require several days to take effect. Immature fetal lungs are more likely to be involved with the newborn respiratory distress syndrome and all its dangers.

○ Rh sensitization. When other evidence of RH sensitization (the Coombs' test, for example) indicate the possibility of progressive fetal involvement and risk, amniotic fluid samples are taken to assess accurately the degree of involvement that exists. Breakdown blood substances in the amniotic fluid can be measured quite accurately and reflect what is happening to the fetal blood system. The test is often used to determine the need for early delivery, or, if the infant is too immature, the need for intrauterine blood transfusions. (See page 122.)

o The need for genetic counseling. (See page 250.)

o Infection. Under certain dangerous circumstances, amniotic fluid may become infected (amnionitis) and threaten fetal existence. Such infection may start from a maternal systemic involvement or from unsuspected and untreated premature rupture of the membranes. Whatever the source, cultures from the amniotic fluid are important in determining the type of infection and the best treatment.

o Premature rupture. Under certain circumstances, premature membrane rupture may be difficult to confirm by the usual methods. A useful technique to help confirm the membrane integrity or lack of it consists of the withdrawal of a small amount of amniotic fluid by amniocentesis, followed by the installation of a harmless dye substance. If the dye shortly appears in vaginal secretions, we have positive proof of premature rupture.

Each year, more fetal secrets are revealed by our ever-widening study of amniotic fluid. It is safe to say that amniocentesis will play an ever-increasing role in the assessment and the management of fetal state.

## FETOLOGY, FETOSCOPY, AND FETAL SURGERY

The new science of fetology continues to wrest more and more secrets from within the developing embryo as a new life begins to weave itself on its magical genetic shuttle. Fetologists are learning ways to enter the uterus with reasonable safety and thus to probe directly at the fetus in order to learn more about its intrauterine growth and development. Moreover, fetologists can now determine the existence of certain intrauterine disorders that can be corrected within the uterus and allow healthy fetal survival.

In order for fetologists to enter the uterine cavity with relative safety, instrumentation had to be developed for that purpose. Thus evolved the fetoscope, a hollow metal tube that could be placed within the uterine cavity and which contains a looking source, a light source, and an operating source. You may have seen somewhat similar instruments used to peer into knee joints (arthroscopes), abdomens (laparoscopes), and bladders (cystoscopes). At any rate, a fetoscope allows direct, if limited, visualization of an intrauterine fetus, with a limited operating capability. Thus, the following may be done:

○ Blood samples may be taken from the placental vessels to detect certain blood disorders such as sickle cell anemia or thalassemia.

○ Skin biopsies may be taken through the operative fetoscope and used in genetic analysis.

○ Muscle biopsies may be taken to reveal certain types of inherited dystrophies.

It must be made clear that fetoscopy is highly investigational and experimental. There are few institutions capable of providing this service at the present time. And there are real risks of infection and of premature labor as a result of this invasive procedure. So the goals must be very well defined indeed.

### Fetal surgery

As a normal consequence of fetoscopy, there has been a developing interest in performing intrauterine fetal surgery to correct conditions that might otherwise destroy the fetus before or during birth. As an example, if hydrocephaly (enlarged fetal head due to excessive spinal fluid accumulation) is present, delivery may be impossible without damaging the infant from the sheer size of its head. By operating within the uterus and decompressing the fetal head from the excessive spinal fluid, the child may be saved. This procedure is being done right now.

Many other forms of fetal surgery are being contemplated or attempted and eventually this will be a recognized, if limited, surgical specialty. In the meantime, progress is slow and limited. Recently, restrictions have been advised for some procedures, but nonetheless, fetal surgery must:

° Be confined to tertiary centers.

° Be performed by fetologists.

° Have available state-of-the-art ultrasound.

° Have available state-of-the-art labor inhibition techniques.

° Have clearly recognized and acceptable fetal goals.

ooooooooooooo **THINGS TO THINK ABOUT** ooooooooooooo

There are at this time 55 million American women of childbearing age, fifteen to forty-four years. Here is their track record:

° Thirty million use some form of contraception, including tubal sterilization.

° Over 5 million have problems with infertility and 20 percent of them seek help for this problem each year.

° There are about 6 million pregnancies each year. At least 15 percent—and probably more—end up aborting spontaneously. Of the remainder, one in four will have an induced abortion.

° In the remaining group, 3.6 million infants will deliver, of which 40,000 will die within one year, usually from problems associated with low birth weight.

° All but 1 percent of the deliveries will be in hospitals and attended by physicians, a relatively constant figure.

° Obstetrical deliveries account for only 4.6 percent of the total hospital days in the United States. This is because hospital confinement after delivery is on the average only about three days.

° The average charge made by a hospital for a normal vaginal delivery in 1982 was $1,130 and for a section, $1,930. The total American cost for delivery services is $8.2 billion each year, of which 60 percent represents hospital charges.

° The average fee for a normal delivery by an obstetrician in 1982 was $700. It is probably now considerably higher as the cost of malpractice insurance soars. In some states $800 has to be added to each doctor's fee to cover malpractice premiums *alone.*

○ The average charge for an anesthesiologist's care at a normal delivery in 1982 was $150 and for a cesarian section, $250.

○ The cost of medical care for babies in their first year of life was $6.5 billion. Only 10 percent of that amount was spent on healthy-baby care. Sixty percent was for newborn care and associated problems and the remaining 30 percent was for subsequent hospitalization during the first year after birth.

○ Pediatric care averaged $64 for a normal newborn and the hospital nursery charges averaged $340. On the other hand, the charges for managing a problem newborn under prolonged intensive care in one study averaged $40,000 and there are cases now that approach $100,000 for such care—a very strong argument for castastrophic insurance protection.

○○○○○○○○

**Lawsuits.** This is an emotionally charged area. We are all now suing the feet out from under each other and the rest of the country is finally feeling the pressure that doctors have felt for years. And so it comes about that liability insurance is being denied or is beyond the financial reach of many American businesses. Moreover, massive damage awards are wiping out whole corporations.

Everyone has and should have the right to seek nonfrivolous redress when they feel that they have been wronged. However, lately the pursuit of a free lunch via the courts has supplanted baseball as the national pastime, has become a career goal to many and a moral obligation to others. But there is no free lunch and so the national lawsuit lottery must soon come to an end.

Obstetricians fear lawsuits just as most everyone else does. Because of the critical nature of our specialty we are prime targets for legal action. At least 70 percent of us have been sued, many more than once. Does this mean that we are that much more stupid or inept than our colleagues thirty years ago who were subject to lawsuits at the rate of about 5 percent? If we are, then why is infant and maternal mortality and morbidity decreasing at its present rapid rate?

Here are some things you may not have considered or know about:

○ Obstetricians' malpractice premiums in some areas of our country are approaching and surpassing $100,000 each year. Obstetricians have no other income than their practices. Where, then, does the money come from for the malpractice premiums? You got it—or you had it, rather. An obstetrician who delivers the usual average of 200 babies per year will have to add at least $500 to your bill for his premiums. And if you feel forced to sue him you will end up, should you win, with about 30 percent of that settlement.

○ The court awards that you read about represent just the tip of the iceberg. Most malpractice money and time is spent in years of pretrial depositions, discovery hearings, and conferences. Probably doctors fear this most of all. The time away from their work, nights of sleeplessness and agonizing, endless hours of legal hassling and delays, depression and loss of confidence—all these things haunt them more than any other one factor.

○ Our self-destructive holster shooting is also forcing many talented, good, and faithful obstetricians to discontinue their work. As follows:

At least 15 percent of all obstetricians in Florida are leaving the field each year.

Rising malpractice insurance has forced all the obstetricians on Molokai Island, Hawaii, to stop delivering babies. Pregnant women on that island now have to be flown to Honolulu for obstetrical care.

In many of our states, obstetricians are beginning to turn away new patients as the fear of lawsuits mounts and malpractice premiums rise. A recent boycott took place in Massachusetts and one is now threatening in Maryland.

○ The insurance companies are not now making a killing. If they were, they would be tumbling all over themselves to get into malpractice coverage. Instead, they are all trying to get out of it. Would you close a successful business?

Obviously, these comments will not solve the American liability crisis, but they may provide you with some food for thought about our future—all of our futures. We may litigate ourselves into oblivion.

○ ○ ○ ○ ○ ○ ○ ○ ○ ○ ○ ○ ○ ○ ○ ○ ○ ○ ○ ○ ○ ○ ○ ○ ○ ○ ○ ○ ○ ○ ○ ○ ○ ○ ○ ○ ○ ○ ○ ○ ○ ○ ○ ○

# ° Conclusion °
# Managing a Primelife Pregnancy

Now that you know the medical and technical facts of primelife pregnancy, it is time to come down on all the things we have been talking about and to outline the typical management of a primelife pregnancy. Please be aware, though, that there may be marked variations of the following protocol because of:

° Different approaches by different obstetricians.

° Local constraining factors. All areas of the United States and other developed countries do not constantly have available certain technical facilities.

° In this rapidly changing field, new procedures may be available that were not known at print time.

° I may have overlooked something.

## PRIMELIFE PROGRAM

### Prepregnancy

It is of value to have an obstetrical consultation many months before pregnancy becomes a fact. At that time, you will have an opportunity to ask questions important to you. Your proposed obstetrician will also have an equal opportunity to lay some advice upon you. Thus you may hear about:

∘ Your diet, which should be patterned after the regular obstetrical diet.

∘ Weight control. Your ideal weight (or the closest you can get to it) should be achieved several months before conception. No weight loss should be contemplated after that time.

∘ A standard vitamin/mineral supplement is indicated.

∘ Vigorous exercise should be avoided. That would include any exercise program designed to significantly raise your pulse, respirations, or body temperatures for any length of time.

∘ All possible medications should be avoided, particularly in the second half of each menstrual cycle.

∘ Tobacco, alcohol, and drugs need to be eliminated. This and many other of these suggestions involve your unimpregnated coconspirator as well.

∘ Medical problems need to be brought under tight control.

### First trimester

The first obstetrical visit should be as early as possible to help date the pregnancy accurately (your last menstrual period is not accurate), to ascertain its health and its location, and, as far as you are concerned, to get a grasp on any complicating medical problem.

Besides the regular history and physical examination and routine complete blood testing (see page 13), special procedures may be ordered.

∘ An ultrasound examination at this time can help date the pregnancy very accurately, and be invaluable for comparison later on. It can also assess the health of an early pregnancy.

∘ Beta HCG pregnancy testing may be done if the pregnancy health is in question. You also know it can offer supportive evidence in the diagnosis of an ectopic pregnancy.

° Certain extra laboratory studies are necessary to assess an ongoing medical problem.

Following all this, you will consult with your doctor about the continuing management of your pregnancy, what you are expected to do, what the doctor is expected to do, and how frequently you need to see each other.

If nothing befalls the pregnancy and you have no complicating medical condition, you will probably have two more regular visits in the first trimester. If you choose to have chorionic villi sampling (CVS, see pages 252–53) and if the test can be done in your locality, it is generally undertaken about the ninth week. If all goes well with it, you will know the genetic health and the sex of your child within a few days time. If you are Rh negative, Rhogam may be given to you after the first test procedure.

## Second trimester

Involving usually the fourteenth to twenty-eighth week, things now begin to pick up somewhat. You are still seeing your obstetrician at monthly intervals, but by the end of this time frame, your visits will be at least every three weeks.

Alpha fetoprotein testing is done about the fifteenth week (see page 253). A maternal blood sample is taken, and if the level of AFP found in the blood sample is abnormal (high or low), certain fetal abnormalities are now searched for. This AFP test is not done as a rule if you are going to have an amniocentesis because the amniocentesis yields the same information more accurately.

Genetic amniocentesis (see pages 250–52) is also planned for the fifteenth week or thereabouts. The withdrawn amniotic fluid is rich in information about the fetus, but unfortunately the results may take three or more weeks to be harvested. This is indeed a trying time for mothers to endure, and, sad to say, has largely been emotionally overlooked by us obstetricians. After the procedure, Rhogam is given to Rh negative mothers.

About the middle of this trimester a blood count is often repeated and if significant anemia is found to be present, extra iron may be needed, given either orally or intramuscularly. If you are Rh negative, a Coombs' test may also be taken at this time, and finally, in some instances, a vaginal culture is also obtained.

Three important procedures are carried out around the twenty-eighth week:

- Rhogam is given to Rh negative women following the evaluation of the Coombs' test.

- Blood is withdrawn after a measured amount of glucose is somehow swallowed. This test determines the possible presence of gestational diabetes. If the results indicate that possibility, a full-scale sugar tolerance test is arranged.

- A biophysical profile is obtained. This is a level II ultrasound procedure (see pages 259–60) and is of incredible value in assessing the fetal state at this critical time. If it scores well, the third trimester often becomes a somewhat more relaxed time.

## Third trimester

Here the whole show comes together and mother and child are before the footlights, under close surveillance almost all the time lest either makes a misstep that could ring down the curtain. Visits here are soon weekly and often closer than that. Although a good biophysical profile at twenty-eight weeks has been reassuring, close observation is still in order, and if the BPP was not normal, then the watch becomes even more meticulous.

Part of the watch system consists of regular fetal heart rate monitoring under stimulation and under stress. Thus, the various tests—nonstress, stress, breast stimulation, further BPPs, and finally, maternal self-monitoring—are called into play at varying intervals to key your doctor into what is going on in the fetal environment.

As term approaches, amniotic fluid samples may be taken to help in the determination of fetal well-being (in Rh disorders, for instance) and to determine fetal lung maturity. Also, in the final weeks regular pelvic examinations may be performed to assess the feasibility of labor induction should it become necessary.

As long as maternal and fetal health remains stable, early pregnancy interruption by cesarian section or labor induction is usually avoided. However, an increasing maternal problem (deteriorating blood sugar control in a diabetic, for example) or an increasing fetal problem with evidence of fetal distress generally mean that the uterus must be evacuated. Thus, if labor is induced, it will be monitored with care from beginning to end, and if section is the selected delivery route, it too will be managed with the greatest care for both participants.

It is becoming clear that no primelife pregnancy, no matter how healthy it may appear, should go more than two weeks post dates, perhaps not even that far. Thus, accurate pregnancy dating is vital and the early testing suggested above is of great importance and value both in the resolution of postdatism as well as other problems throughout pregnancy. At any rate, primelife mothers who do indeed meet and pass their due dates must be watched with extra devotion and delivered at the earliest safe time, but not later than two weeks after the true expected date.

What has gone before is a standard outline for the management of a high-risk pregnancy. Remember that the disclaimers laid down at the beginning of this segment should always be applied to any individual case. The cutting edge of our knowledge is moving swiftly in this highly sensitive area of maternal care and the written word can rarely chronicle current advances. This means your own obstetrician is farther into the forefront than this book, and procedures that he uses which diverge from this written text are probably superior to it.

We have come to the end of our book and our journey together although you may still be working your way through your much more personal and exciting experience—your primelife pregnancy. True, it may be accompanied by some danger but only enough danger to give the experience some spice and tingle. No matter where in your pregnancy you now find yourself, you are still at the beginning of your total reproductive experience, for it encompasses not only your pregnancy but all that follows as your baby grows and its life unfolds.

Management seminars tell us that problems make opportunities. If primelife pregnancy is a problem, then it is one of the few that will ever offer you so many opportunities for growth, self-understanding, fulfillment, and rewards. And all with limited risk.

Make it work.

# Index

fetus *(cont.)*
259–60; death of, 28–29; and
diabetes of mother, 218; as graft,
24, 27, 32–33; legal rights of, 108–9;
lung maturity, 133, 135; and
maternal malnutrition, 48;
monitoring of, 257–73; and
smoking, 63; surgery of, 273–74
fever, after delivery, 185
fiber, dietary, 102
fibroid tumors of uterus, 199–200
first trimester of pregnancy, 65, 68–69,
279–80; rubella in, 127; TORCH
diseases, 124; travel, 82
fish, as pets, 44
fishing, 39–40
fleas, 43
fluids, in diet, 102
Foley catheters, 177
folic acid, 47, 231–32
folic acid antagonist, 66
follicular stimulating hormone (FSH),
193
food, 49–50, 71; after delivery, 177–78;
in travel, 84. *See also* diet
forceps, 169–71
foreplay, 56–57, 95
formaldehyde, 19
fraternal twins, 119; abortion of one,
214
freezing of chromosomes, 249
frozen embryos, 33
frozen foods, 49
FSH (follicular stimulating hormone),
193

gardening, 42
Gatorade, 84
general anesthesia, 141, 163–64
genes, 116, 249
genetics, 115–16, 206, 249–50; defects,
and age, 194
genital herpes. *See* herpes virus II
German measles. *See* rubella
germ cells, 193–94
gestational diabetes, 218, 220–21; test
for, 281
girdles, 89
glucose tolerance test, 220–21
gonadotropin, 114
gonorrhea, 98, 195, 196
gravity-parity, 172

grief, after abortion, 29, 208–9
guidelines: for alcohol use, 64–65;
employment in pregnancy, 20, 22;
immunizations, 74–79

habit, 62, 202
habitual abortion, 209
hair, in pregnancy, 52
halogenated hydrocarbons, 19
hands, numbness of, 87
hazardous materials, and work, 19
HCG (human chorionic
gonadotropin), 8, 9–10, 244–46
headaches, 93–94; after spinal
anesthetics, 165
health assessment of pregnancy,
244–77
health care spending, 241–42
heart, fetal, monitoring, 261–63
heart attacks, 63
heartburn, 86–87, 104
heart disease, 18, 229–31, 256
heart rate, maternal, 36, 37
heart transplants, 242
heat loss, 36
heavy metals, 19
height and weight tables, 46
help, after delivery, 181
hemoglobin C (HGB C) tests, 271
hemolytic anemia, 232
hemophilia, 250
hemorrhoids, 101, 102–3, 175
hepatitis B, 76, 80, 124, 254; and
breast feeding, 143
heredity, 115–16. *See also* genetics
herpes gestationis, 92
herpes virus II, 99–101, 124, 128, 137,
196–97, 254; in utero exposure, 242
HGB C (hemoglobin C) tests, 271
high blood pressure. *See*
hypertension
high forceps delivery, 170
HLA, and spontaneous abortion, 207
hobbies, 40–42
Hodgkin's disease, 233
home, work at, 23
home care, after delivery, 179–83
home deliveries, 213
hormones, 7–8, 91; placental, 114
hospitals, 12, 112–13, 158–60, 240;
admission for delivery, 149–50; and
cesarian sections, 137–39; delivery

labor, 111, 112, 153–56, 160–61; anesthesia, 161–67; and asthma, 224; delivery aids, 169–72; and diabetes, 219; episiotomy, 167–69; false, 156–57; history of, and exercise, 38; hospital procedures, 158–60; induced, 151–53, 281–82; position for, 186–87; premature, 131–33; prolonged, 157–58; *See also* delivery

lactation, 47

lactic acid, 35; in vaginal secretions, 95

lactoferrin, 143

Lamaze method, 110–11

lamb, and toxoplasmosis, 125

laparascope, 205–6

lawsuits, 275–77

lead, 19

learning disabilities, 63

left side, lying on, 120, 166

legal aspects of pregnancy, 108–9

leg cramps, 85–86

legumes, 50

liability insurance, 275–77

ligament pain, 27

lindane, 19

lithium, 67

live virus vaccines, 73, 74–75

local anesthesia, 55, 164–65

lochia, 176, 182

loperamide (Imodium), 84

loss of pregnancy, 28–29, 31

low birth weight, 128–30, 145–46; death rate, 274

low forceps delivery, 170–71

lung cancer, 63, 233

lung disorders, 222–26

lung maturity of fetus, 271

Lyme disease, 43

macrosomia, 173–74, 218, 220, 242

magnesium sulfate, 132

magnetic resonance imaging, 261

male births. *See* boy babies

male fertility, 196, 202

malnutrition, 31, 48, 131

malpractice insurance, 12, 274–76

mammography, 13, 144, 186, 233

masturbation, 57

maternal blood tests for fetal state, 270–71

maternal deaths, 213–14

maternal self-monitoring, 269–70

maternity clothes, 58–61

maternity leave, 21, 23, 183

measles (rubeola), 74, 81

meats, 49, 50

median episiotomy, 167

medical care costs, 274–75

medical complications of pregnancy, 217–43

medications, 25, 55, 66, 230, 279; while breast feeding, 182; and fertility, 201

mediolateral episiotomy, 167

melanoma, 233

membranes, rupture of, 38, 153–54; in induced labor, 152; premature, 97, 99, 134–35, 137, 272

men: false pregnancy, 28; participation in labor, 111–12; threats to fertility, 212

Mendel, Gregor Johann, 116

meningococcus, 78

menopause, 63, 193, 195

menstruation, missed, 8

mental retardation, 64

meprobamate, 67

mercury, 19, 67

methoxyflurane, 19

metronidazole, 97

microwave radiation, 211

midforceps delivery, 170

migraine headaches, 93

milk, in diet, 50–51, 86, 198

miscarriage, 28–29. *See also* abortion

missed abortion, 20, 208

mitral valve prolapse, 231

monitored labor, 160–61

multiple pregnancies, 38, 115, 118–20, 137, 249

mumps, 74, 124, 126, 242, 254

muscle biopsies, fetal, 273

mycoplasmosis, 98–99

myomectomy, 200

nausea, 8, 24–25, 31–32

necrotizing enterocolitis, 142

neonatology, 239

neurological headaches, 93

newborns, 70, 187–88; and maternal health problems, 98, 99, 100–101, 124–28, 218, 220, 224, 236

NGU (nongonococcal urethritis). *See* chlamydia

Ultrasound *(cont.)*
  membranes, 134; and sex of
    child, 118
umbilical cord, 113, 134, 260
umbilical hernia, 88
underweight, 38, 45, 47, 70
United States government, and infant
    mortality, 147–48
university teaching hospitals, 139–40
unstable joints, 87–88
ureters, in pregnancy, 226
urination, frequent, 8
urine tests, 9–10, 13, 227
uterine contractions, 154–56, 158;
    afterpains, 176; monitoring of, 263,
    265, 266; oxytocin stress test, 267
uterine cramps, 27
uterus, 9; diseases of, 199–200;
    malformation, 131

vaccinations. *See* immunizations
vacuum extraction, 171–72
vaginal bleeding, 29, 30, 38
vaginal douching, 53
vaginal flow, after delivery, 185
vaginal infections, 95–101
vaginal secretions, 132, 153, 176
vaginitis, 60
Valsalva maneuver, 36
varicella (chicken pox), 77, 124, 254
varicose veins, 91
VDT (video display terminal), 211
veins, dilated, 91

venereal diseases. *See* sexually
    transmitted diseases
vibrations, 211
video display terminal (VDT), 211
vinyl chloride, 19
viruses, exposure to, 19; in utero
    exposure, 242
vitamin/mineral supplements, 24, 47,
    48, 54, 92, 182, 232
vitamins, 67, 234–35; B6, for nausea,
    25; K, and epilepsy, 234–35
vomiting, 24–25, 31–32, 234; after
    anesthesia, 164; and tooth decay,
    54

waistline in maternity clothes, 59
warfarin, 66
warts, vaginal, 99
Wass, D. M., 254
water sports, 40
weight, 45–48, 92; prepregnancy, 279
women: infection with AIDS, 237;
    resident physicians, low birth
    weight babies, 146
work, 17–24; after delivery, 182–83
worms, of dogs, 43

x-rays, 55, 201–2

yeast infections, 53, 60, 96–97
yellow fever, 75

zinc, 47

## ABOUT THE AUTHOR

Dr. Gillespie was born in North Bay, Ontario, Canada, and educated at McGill University in Montreal. His training in obstetrics and gynecology was completed in the United States and he now lives and practices in Little Rock, Arkansas. Dr. Gillespie is certified by the American Board of Obstetrics and Gynecology and is a Fellow of the American College of Obstetricians and Gynecologists. In 1977 he was elected a Fellow of the Royal College of Obstetricians and Gynecologists in London, England, an unusual honor for American citizens. Besides his private practice he serves as clinical professor of obstetrics and gynecology at the University of Arkansas School of Medicine. He is a member of a number of scientific societies and has received awards for his research from the American Medical Association, the Southern Medical Association, the American Fertility Society, and the Pacific Coast Fertility Society.

Dr. Gillespie is the author of numerous scientific publications, as well as *Your Pregnancy Month by Month* (third edition, Harper & Row).